Sirtfood Cookbook for Women Over 40

Delicious Recipes To Lead A Healthy And Balanced Life

By Miguel Gutierrez

1

Sommario

Introduction

The Sirtfood diet plan, well-known amongst the VIPs as the "lean genetics" diet regimen, bases its efficiency on boosting the sirtuins by eating details foods. The sirtuins can melt fat swiftly as well as without calling for unneeded sacrifices. The Sirt Diet regimen changes not eating with a cautious option of foods. It includes 2 unique stages, the initial stage, which lasts one week, is for fat loss, and also the 2nd stage, which lasts 2 weeks, is for weight upkeep.

With this diet plan, you can melt 3 kg in a week without making considerable initiatives. Light exercise is advised, as well as we suggest seeking advice from a medical professional to make a correct diet regimen strategy.

In this publication, you will certainly discover delicious dishes, train on your own to prepare them; some will certainly need to be done a number of times to obtain the very best outcome.

Effort does not terrify you, and also consuming purposely is an objective we need to all pursue. Great.

Chapter 1 Breakfast Recipes

Cherry Tomatoes Red Pesto Porridge

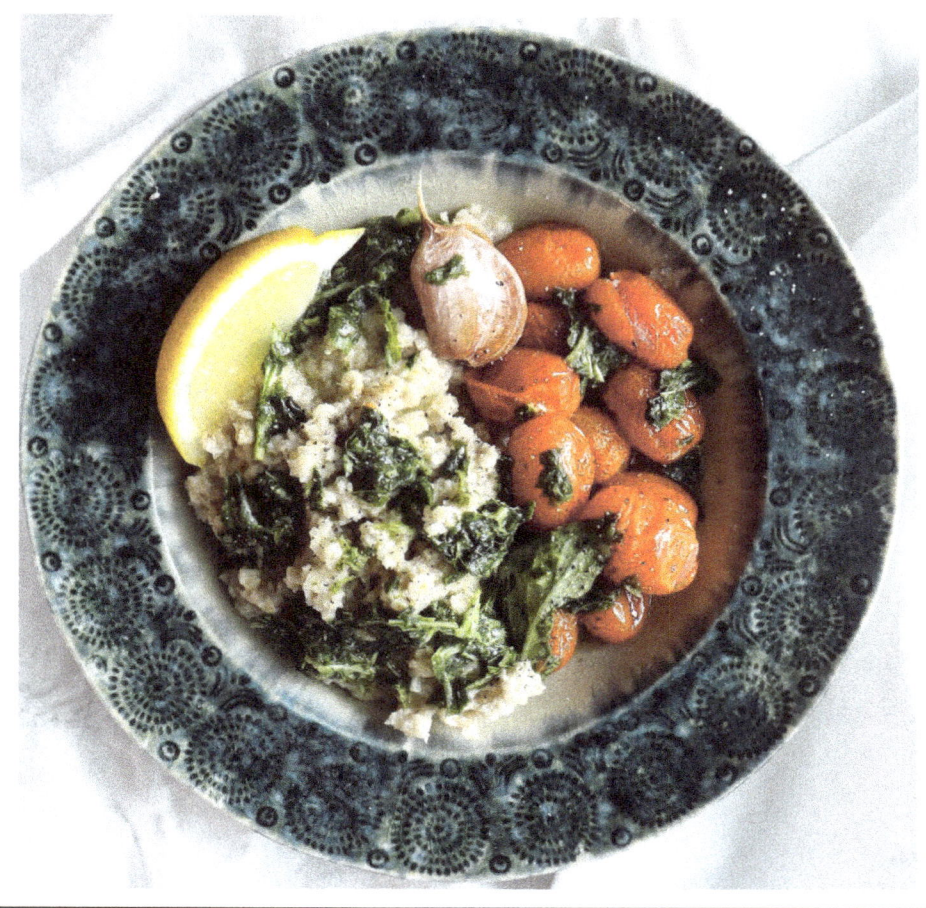

Preparation Time: 10 minutes
Cooking Time: 5 minutes
Servings: 2

INGREDIENTS:

Salt, pepper 1 teaspoon hemp seed 1 teaspoon pumpkin seed

2 teaspoons nutritional yeast ½ cup couscous ½ cup oats

1 teaspoon sun-dried tomato-walnut pesto 1 teaspoon tahini

1 tablespoon callion 1 cup sliced cherry tomatoes 1 cup chopped kale

1 teaspoon dried basil 1.5 teaspoon dried oregano 2 cups veggie stock

Directions:

In a small cooking pot, add oats, oregano, vegetable stock, basil, couscous, pepper and salt and cook for about 5 minutes on medium heat stirring frequently until porridge is creamy and soft.

Add chopped kale but reserve a bit for garnish, tomatoes and sliced scallion. Cook for additional 1 minute, stir in pesto, tahini, and nutritional yeast. Top with the reserved kale, pumpkin and hemp seeds plus cherry tomatoes.

Nutrition:

Calories: 259 Net carbs: 36g Fat: 7.68g Fiber: 7.4g Protein: 14.26g

Sautéed Veggies Bowl

Preparation time: 5 minutes
Cooking time: 5 minutes
Servings: 1

INGREDIENTS:

For tofu scramble:

1 cup water

Dash of soy sauce

Pepper and salt

1 teaspoon turmeric

1 serving medium crumbled firm tofu

For the Sautéed Veggies:

1/2 cup red onions, diced

1 cup mushrooms, sliced

1 big handful kale, de-stemmed and chopped

For the Bowls

1/2 cup cooked brown rice

1/2 avocado, pitted

Directions:

Mix together the tofu scramble ingredients in a small dish, set aside.

Add a splash of water in a skillet over medium-high heat; add the onions, mushrooms and kale. Cook, stirring periodically, for about 5-8 minutes or until it is evenly brown and soft. Set aside in a bowl.

Using the same skillet, pour in the tofu mixture and cook until it starts to brown and heated through for 5 minutes.

Transfer tofu scramble into a bowl, add the mushrooms/kale mixture, top with avocado, brown rice and salsa. Serve with flatbreads, buckwheat, basmati rice or couscous.

Nutrition:

Calories: 122g

Fats: 6.9g

Sodium 867g

Net carbs: 8.7g

Fiber: 1.7g

Sugar: 4.9g

Protein: 7.3g

Chocolate Oats Granola

Preparation time: 10 minutes
Cooking time: 20 minutes
Servings: 8

INGREDIENTS:

60 grams good-quality dark chocolate chips (70%)

2 of rice malt syrup or maple syrup

1 tablespoon dark brown sugar

20g roughly chopped butter

3 teaspoons light olive oil

50g roughly chopped pecans

200g of jumbo oats

Directions:

Heat-up your oven to 160°C).

In a large bowl, mix together pecan and oats. Gently heat the butter, olive oil, rice malt syrup and brown sugar in a small non-stick pan until the sugar and syrup is dissolved and butter melted. Do not allow the mixture boil before removing. Spread the mixture on top the oats and stir very well to coat with the oats.

Distribute the oats mixture onto a large parchment lined baking tray, spread out into every corners. You do not need to spread evenly, leave lumps of mixture with spacing.

Place tray in the oven and bake until edges are just tinged golden brown, about 20 minutes. Withdraw from the oven and let completely cool on the tray.

Once cool, use your finger to break up any lager lumps. Add in the chocolate chips and mix. Serve Chocolate granola with cup of green tea.

Nutrition:

Calories: 244

Net carbs: 20.91g

Fat: 15.41g

Fiber: 4.6 g

Protein: 5.24g

Green Chia Spinach Pudding

Preparation Time: 30 minutes
Cooking Time: 0 minutes
Servings: 1

INGREDIENTS:

3 spoons of chia seeds 1 Medjool date, slice in half and remove pit

1 handful fresh spinach 1 cup non-dairy milk Toppings

Banana, berries, etc.

Directions:

Blend the spinach, date and milk in a high speed blender until very smooth.

Pour the mixture in a bowl over the chia seeds. Stir mixture well, and stirring every now and then for about 15 minutes.

Transfer to the fridge and allow to chill at least one hour or overnight.

Stir once more, just before serving; top with kiwi, banana, berries, etc.

Nutrition:

Calories: 232g Fats: 9.6g Sodium 86mg Net Carbs: 2.6g

Fiber: 9.9g Protein 10.1g

Blackcurrant and Raspberry Breakfast

Preparation time: 5 minutes
Cooking time: 15 minutes
Servings: 2

INGREDIENTS:

300 ml water 2 teaspoons granulated sugar

100 grams blackcurrants, washed and stalks removed 2 leaves gelatin

100 grams raspberries, washed

Directions:

In two serving glasses, add the raspberries and set aside.

Add cold water in a bowl and place the gelatin leaves to soften.

In a small pan, add the blackcurrants with 100 ml of water along with the sugar. Bring to the boil. Let it simmer for five minutes and then turn heat off. Remove and cool for 2 minutes.

Remove the gelatin leaves and squeeze out excess water. Place leaves in the saucepan. Stir constantly until completely dissolved, add in the remaining water and stir together. Pour liquid over raspberries in the glasses or dishes. Place in the refrigerator for about 3-4 hours or overnight and allow to set.

Nutrition:

Calories: 76 Net carbs: 13.57g Fat: 0.5g Fiber: 3.3 g Protein: 4g

Kale Mushroom Scramble

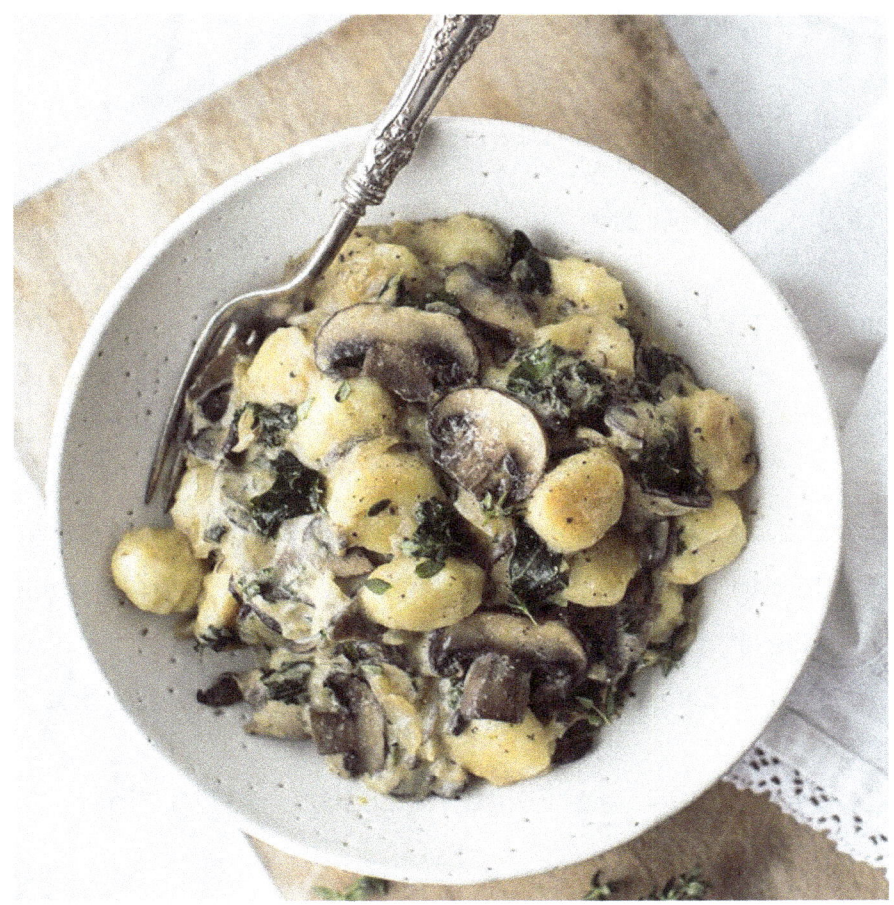

Preparation time: 10 minutes
Cooking time: 6 minutes
Servings: 1

INGREDIENTS:

5g of finely chopped parsley

Handful of thinly sliced button mushrooms

½ thinly sliced bird's eye chili

1 teaspoon extra virgin olive oil

20g kale, roughly chopped

1 teaspoon mild curry powder

1 teaspoon ground turmeric 2 eggs

Directions:

Mix together the curry powder, turmeric and a small splash of water to form a light paste. Add the kale to a steamer basket and steam in boiling water for 2– 3 minutes. Heat the oil over medium heat in a frying pan and fry mushrooms and chili for 2 to 3 minutes until soften and starting to brown.

Nutrition: Calories: 116g Fats: 5.4g Net carbs: 13.2g Fiber: 3.6g Proteins 5.8g

Walnut Medjool Porridge

Preparation time: 10 minutes
Cooking time: 15 minutes
Servings: 1

INGREDIENTS:

50g strawberries, hulled

1 teaspoon walnut butter

35g Buckwheat flakes

1 chopped Medjool date

200 ml almond or coconut milk, unsweetened

Directions:

Add the date and milk into a frying pan over medium low heat, then add in the flakes and cook to your desired consistency.

Add in the walnut butter, stir well. Top porridge with strawberries.

Nutrition:

Calories: 550 Net carbs: 25g Fat: 45g Fiber: 9 g Protein: 6.57g

Avocado Tofu Breakfast Salad

Preparation Time: 5 minutes
Cooking time: 5 minutes
Servings: 1

INGREDIENTS:

Half a lemon juice Half a red onion, chopped 2 tomatoes, chopped

One spoon chili sauce 4 handfuls baby spinach

A handful of chopped almonds 1 pink chopped grapefruit

1 Avocado, chopped Half a pack of firm tofu, chopped 2 Tortillas

Directions:

Heat the tortillas in the oven for 8 to 10 minutes.

Combine tomatoes, tofu and onions with some chili sauce in a bowl, place inside the refrigerator to cool.

Add the avocado, grapefruit and almonds. Mix everything together and place into the bowl.

Top with a Squeeze of fresh lemon juice!

Nutrition:

Calories 94g Fats 2.1g Net Carbs 11.3gProtein 3.9g

Buckwheat Coconut Overnight Porridge

Preparation time: 10 minutes
Cooking time: 8 minutes
Servings: 4-6

INGREDIENTS:

1/4 teaspoon of cinnamon 2 teaspoon of vanilla extract 1 cup water

3 cups unsweetened coconut, soy or almond milk 1/4 cup chia seeds

1 cup of buckwheat groats (not kasha) Pinch of salt

For the Toppings:

1 1/2 cup berries 1/2 cup walnuts

Directions:

In a bowl, combine together the buckwheat groats, coconut milk, chia seeds, cinnamon, water, vanilla extract and salt. Cover bowl with stretch film, transfer to the fridge and let sit overnight.

Bring it out in the morning and place it in a pot; cook mixture in the pot for 10-12 minutes, stirring occasionally until your desired thickness is reached. Add the toppings and Serve.

Nutrition:

Calories: 400 Net carbs: 47g Fat: 17.55g Fiber: 3.7g Protein: 11.19g

Strawberry and Cherry Smoothie

Preparation time: 10 minutes
Cooking time: 0 minutes
Servings: 1

Ingredients:

100g strawberries

75g frozen pitted cherries

1 cup plain full-fat yogurt

175mls unsweetened soya milk

Directions:

Place all of the ingredients into a blender and process until smooth.

Nutrition:

Calories: 132

Fats: 1.5g

Net Carbs: 28.4g

Fiber: 2.9g

Proteins 2.9g

Banana Snap

Preparation time: 10 minutes
Cooking time: 0 minutes
Servings: 1

Ingredients:

2.5cm chunk fresh ginger, peeled 1 banana 1 large carrot

1 apple, cored ½ stick of celery ¼ level teaspoon turmeric powder

Directions:

Place all the ingredients into a blender with just enough water to cover them. Process until smooth

Nutrition:

Calories: 34 Net carbs: 7.8g Fat: 0.1g Fiber: 3.7g Protein: 2g

Green Egg Scramble

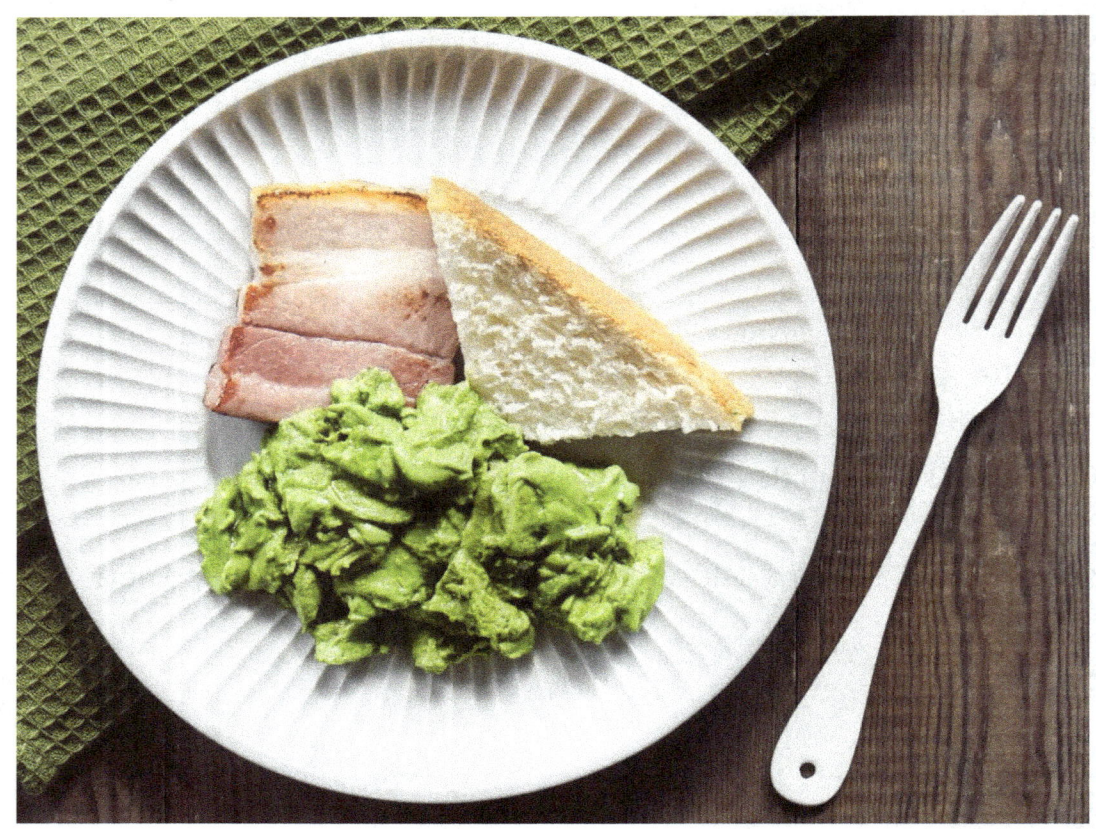

Preparation time: 5 minutes
Cooking time: 5 minutes
Servings: 1

Ingredients:

2 eggs, whisked

25g rocket (arugula) leaves

10g chives, chopped

10g teaspoon fresh basil, chopped

10g teaspoon fresh parsley, chopped

1 teaspoon olive oil

Directions:

Mix the eggs together with the rocket (arugula) and herbs. Heat the oil in a frying pan and pour into the egg mixture. Gently stir until it's lightly scrambled. Season and serve.

Nutrition:

Calories: 101 Net carbs: 2.1g Fat: 7g Fiber: 0.5g Protein: 7.1g

Green Sirtfood Smoothie

Preparation time: 10 minutes
Cooking time: 0 minutes
Servings: 1

Ingredients: 100g unsweetened Greek yoghurt 6 walnut halves

8-10 medium strawberries A handful of kale leaves

20g dark chocolate (min. 85% cocoa) 1 date 1/2 teaspoon turmeric

Small piece fresh chili, finely chopped

200ml unsweetened almond milk

Directions: Put everything into a blender and mix until you get a smoothie.

Nutrition: Calories: 72 Net carbs: 14g Fat: 0.3g Fiber: 0.8g

Protein: 2.8g

Chapter 2 Lunch Recipes

Coq Au Vin

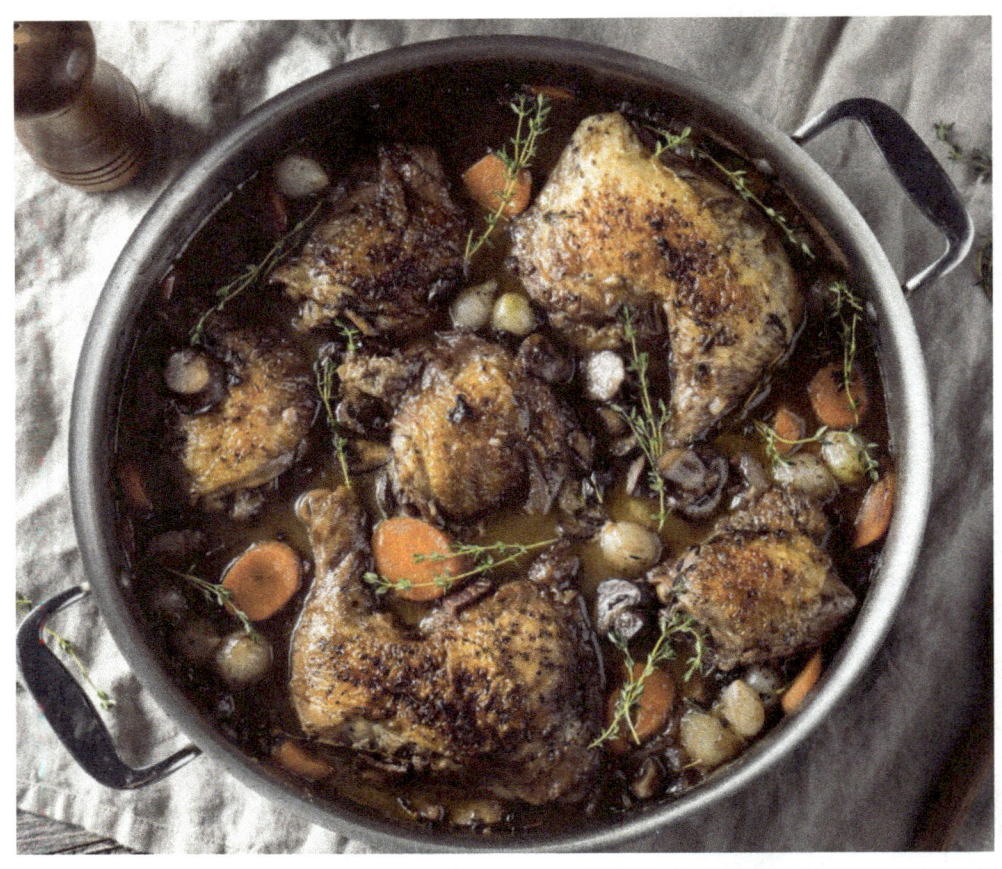

Preparation time: 15 minutes
Cooking time: 1 hour 15 minutes
Servings: 8

Ingredients:

450g button mushrooms

100g streaky bacon, chopped

16 chicken thighs, skin removed

3 cloves of garlic, crushed

3g fresh parsley, chopped

3 carrots, chopped

2 red onions, chopped

2 tablespoons plain flour

2 teaspoons olive oil

750mls red wine

1 bouquet garnish

Directions:

Place the flour on a large plate and coat the chicken in it. Heat the olive oil in a large saucepan, add the chicken and brown it, before setting aside. Fry the bacon in the pan then add the onion and cook for 5 minutes. Pour in the red wine and add the chicken, carrots, bouquet garnish and garlic. Transfer it to a large ovenproof dish. Cook in the oven at 180C/360F for 1 hour. Remove the bouquet garnish and skim off any excess fat, if necessary. Add in the mushrooms and cook for 15 minutes. Stir in the parsley just before serving.

Nutrition:

Calories: 459

Net carbs: 66g

Fat: 1g

Fiber: 4g8g

Turkey Satay Skewers

Preparation time: 10 minutes
Cooking time: 10 minutes
Servings: 2

Ingredients:

250g turkey breast, cubed

25g smooth peanut butter

1 clove of garlic, crushed

½ small bird's eye chili (or more if you like it hotter), finely chopped

½ teaspoon ground turmeric

200mls coconut milk

2 teaspoons soy sauce

Directions:

Combine the coconut milk, peanut butter, turmeric, soy sauce, garlic and chili. Add the turkey pieces to the bowl and stir them until they are completely coated. Push the turkey onto metal skewers. Place the satay skewers on a barbeque or under a hot grill (broiler) and cook for 4-5 minutes on each side, until they are completely cooked.

Nutrition:

Calories: 431 Fat: 0.9g Protein: 4g

Salmon and Capers

Preparation time: 10 minutes
Cooking time: 5 minutes
Servings: 4

Ingredients:

75g Greek yogurt

4 salmon fillets, skin removed

4 teaspoons Dijon Mustard

1 capers, chopped

2 teaspoons fresh parsley

Zest of 1 lemon

Directions:

In a bowl, mix together the yogurt, mustard, lemon zest, parsley and capers. Thoroughly coat the salmon in the mixture. Place the salmon under a hot grill (broiler) and cook for 3-4 minutes on each side, or until the fish is cooked. Serve with mashed potatoes and vegetables or a large green leafy salad.

Nutrition:

Calories: 321

Fat: 6.7g

Protein: 24.5g

Moroccan Chicken Casserole

Preparation time: 20 minutes
Cooking time: 50 minutes
Servings: 4

Ingredients: 4 chicken breasts, cubed

250g tinned chickpeas (garbanzo beans) drained

4 medjool dates, halved

6 dried apricots, halved

1 red onion, sliced 1 carrot, chopped

1 teaspoon ground cumin

1 teaspoon ground cinnamon

1 teaspoon ground turmeric

1 bird's-eye chili, chopped

600mls chicken stock

25g corn flour 60mls water

2 teaspoons fresh coriander

Directions:

Place the chicken, chickpeas (garbanzo beans), onion, carrot, chili, cumin, turmeric, cinnamon and stock (broth) into a large saucepan. Bring it to the boil, reduce the heat and simmer for 25 minutes. Add in the dates and apricots and simmer for 10 minutes. In a cup, mix the corn flour together with the water until it becomes a smooth paste. Pour the mixture into the saucepan and stir until it thickens. Add in the coriander (cilantro) and mix well. Serve with buckwheat or couscous.

Nutrition: Calories: 401 Net carbs: 3.6g

Fat: 4.8g Fiber: 1.7g Protein: 29.2g

Prawn and Coconut Curry

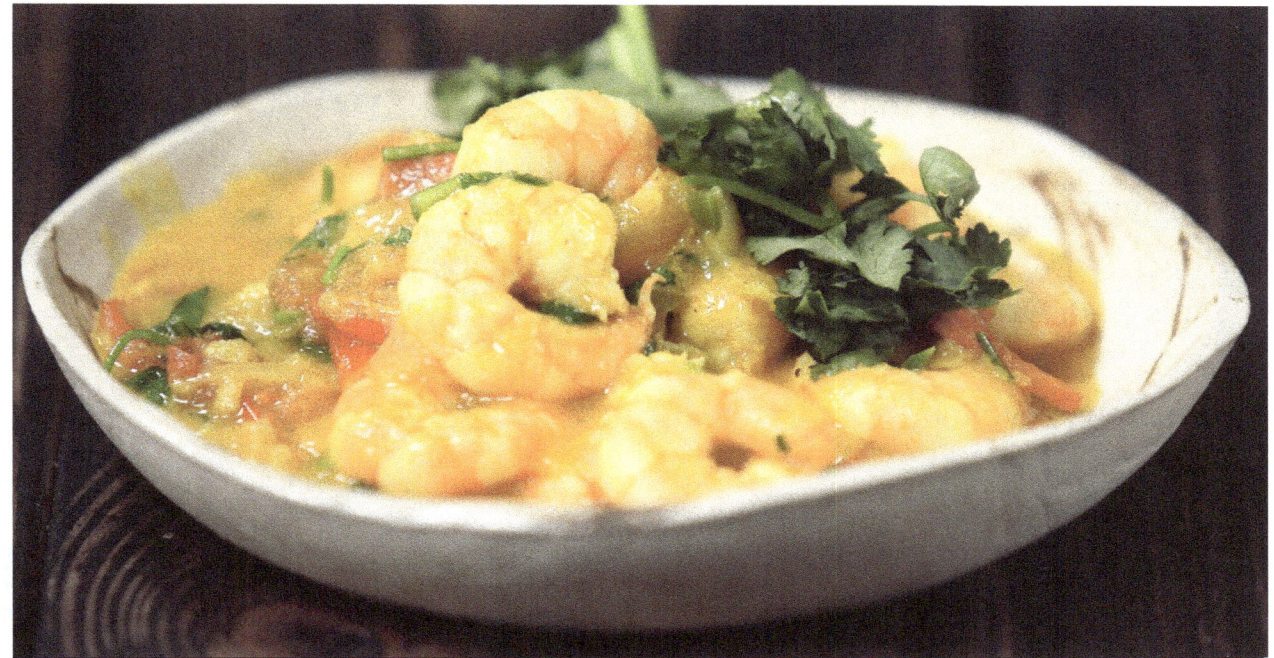

Preparation time: 10 minutes
Cooking time: 5 minutes
Servings: 4

Ingredients:

400g tinned chopped tomatoes

400g large prawns (shrimps), shelled and raw

25g fresh coriander (cilantro) chopped

3 red onions, finely chopped

3 cloves of garlic, crushed

2 bird's eye chilies

½ teaspoon ground coriander (cilantro)

½ teaspoon turmeric

400mls (14fl Oz) coconut milk

1 teaspoons olive oil

Juice of 1 lime

Directions:

Place the onions, garlic, tomatoes, chilies, lime juice, turmeric, ground coriander (cilantro), chilies and half of the fresh coriander (cilantro) into a blender and blitz until you have a smooth curry paste. Heat the olive oil in a frying pan, add the paste and cook for 2 minutes. Stir in the coconut milk and warm it thoroughly. Add the prawns (shrimps) to the paste and cook them until they have turned pink and are completely cooked. Stir in the fresh coriander (cilantro). Serve with rice.

Nutrition: Calories: 322 Net carbs: 98.9g

Fat: 11.8g Fiber: 8g Protein: 15.6g

Chicken and Bean Casserole

Preparation time: 15 minutes
Cooking time: 55 minutes
Servings: 4

Ingredients:

400g chopped tomatoes

400g tinned cannellini beans or haricot beans

8 chicken thighs, skin removed

2 carrots, peeled and finely chopped

2 red onions, chopped

4 sticks of celery

4 large mushrooms

2 red peppers (bell peppers), de-seeded and chopped

1 clove of garlic

2 teaspoons soy sauce

1 olive oil

1.75 liters chicken stock (broth)

Directions:

Heat the olive oil in a saucepan, add the garlic and onions and cook for 5 minutes. Add in the chicken and cook for 5 minutes then add the carrots, cannellini beans, celery, red peppers (bell peppers) and mushrooms. Pour in the stock (broth) soy sauce and tomatoes. Bring it to the boil, reduce the heat and simmer for 45 minutes. Serve with rice or new potatoes.

Nutrition: Calories: 509 Net carbs: 12.5g

Fat: 6.5g Fiber: 1.1g Protein: 27.4g

Mussels in Red Wine Sauce

Preparation time: 5 minutes
Cooking time: 5 minutes
Servings: 2

Ingredients:

800g mussels

2 x 400g tins of chopped tomatoes

25g butter

1 fresh chives, chopped

1 fresh parsley, chopped

1 bird's-eye chili, finely chopped

4 cloves of garlic, crushed

400mls red wine

Juice of 1 lemon

Directions:

Wash the mussels, remove their beards and set them aside. Heat the butter in a large saucepan and add in the red wine. Reduce the heat and add the parsley, chives, chili and garlic whilst stirring. Add in the tomatoes, lemon juice and mussels. Cover the saucepan and cook for 2-3.Remove the saucepan from the heat and take out any mussels which haven't opened and discard them. Serve and eat immediately.

Nutrition:

Calories: 364

Net carbs: 3.3g Fat: 4.9g Fiber: 0.7g

Protein: 8.2g

Roast Balsamic Vegetables

Preparation time: 10 minutes
Cooking time: 45 minutes
Servings: 4

Ingredients:

4 tomatoes, chopped 2 red onions, chopped

3 sweet potatoes, peeled and chopped

100g red chicory (or if unavailable, use yellow)

100g kale, finely chopped

300g potatoes, peeled and chopped

5 stalks of celery, chopped

1 bird's-eye chili, de-seeded and finely chopped

2g fresh parsley, chopped

2gs fresh coriander (cilantro) chopped

3 teaspoons olive oil

2 teaspoons balsamic vinegar

1 teaspoon mustard Sea salt

Freshly ground black pepper

Directions:

Place the olive oil, balsamic, mustard, parsley and coriander (cilantro) into a bowl and mix well. Toss all the remaining ingredients into the dressing and season with salt and pepper. Transfer the vegetables to an ovenproof dish and cook in the oven at 200C/400F for 45 minutes.

Nutrition: Calories: 310 Net carbs: 1.1g

Fiber: 0.2g Protein: 0.2g

Tomato and Goat's Pizza

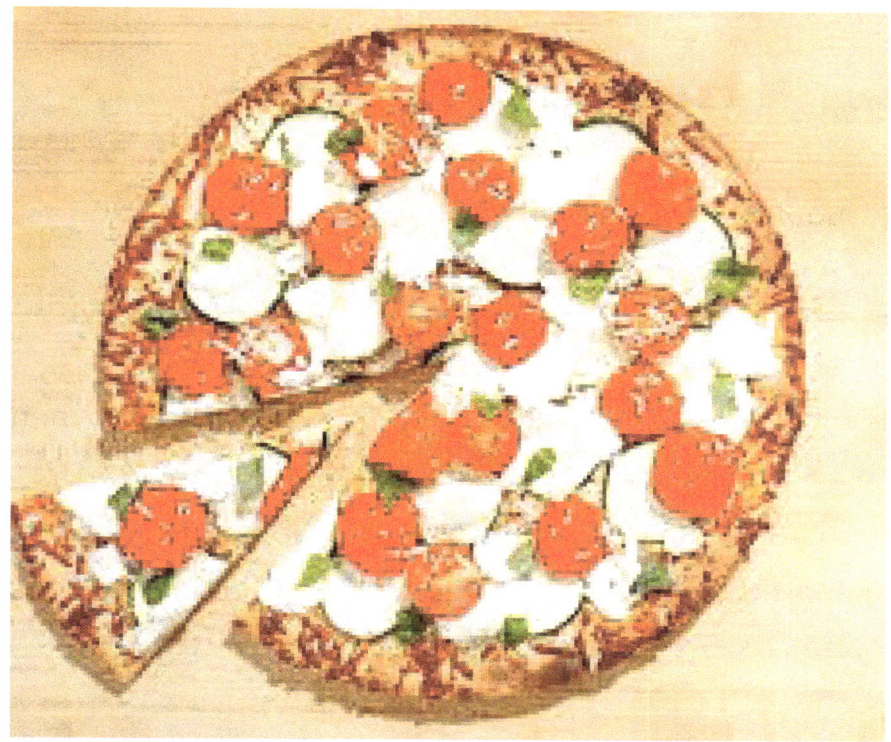

Preparation time: 15 minutes
Cooking time: 20 minutes
Servings: 2

Ingredients: 225g buckwheat flour

2 teaspoons dried yeast Pinch of salt

150mls slightly water 1 teaspoon olive oil

For the Topping:

75g feta cheese, crumbled

75g peseta (or tomato paste)

1 tomato, sliced 1 red onion, finely chopped

25g rocket (arugula) leaves, chopped

Directions:

In a bowl, combine all the ingredients for the pizza dough then allow it to stand for at least an hour until it has doubled in size. Roll the dough out to a size to suit you. Spoon the passata onto the base and add the rest of the toppings. Bake in the oven at 200C/400F for 15-20 minutes or until browned at the edges and crispy and serve.

Nutrition:

Calories: 585 Net carbs: 77g Fat: 8.1g

Fiber: 7.6g Protein: 22.9g

Tender Spiced Lamb

Preparation time: 20 minutes
Cooking time: 4 hours 20 minutes
Servings: 8

Ingredients:

1.35kg lamb shoulder

3 red onions, sliced

3 cloves of garlic, crushed

1 bird's eye chili, finely chopped

1 teaspoon turmeric

1 teaspoon ground cumin

½ teaspoon ground coriander (cilantro)

¼ teaspoon ground cinnamon

2 tablespoons olive oil

Directions:

In a bowl, combine the chili, garlic and spices with olive oil. Coat the lamb with the spice mixture and marinate it for an hour, or overnight if you can. Heat the remaining oil in a pan, add the lamb and brown it for 3-4 minutes on all sides to seal it. Place the lamb in an ovenproof dish. Add in the red onions and cover the dish with foil. Transfer to the oven and roast at 170C/325F for 4 hours. The lamb should be extremely tender and falling off the bone. Serve with rice or couscous, salad or vegetables.

Nutrition:

Calories: 455 Net carbs: 28g

Fat: 9.8g Fiber: 11g Protein: 20g

Chili Cod Fillets

Preparation time: 10 minutes
Cooking time: 10 minutes
Servings: 4

Ingredients:

4 cod fillets each)

2 teaspoons fresh parsley, chopped

2 bird's-eye chilies (or more if you like it hot)

2 cloves of garlic, chopped

4 teaspoons olive oil

Directions:

Heat a of olive oil in a frying pan, add the fish and cook for 7-8 minutes or until thoroughly cooked, turning once halfway through. Remove and keep warm. Pour the remaining olive oil into the pan and add the chili, chopped garlic and parsley. Warm it thoroughly. Serve the fish onto plates and pour the warm chili oil over it.

Nutrition:

Calories: 246 Net carbs: 5.5g

Fat: 0.5g Fiber: 0.7g Protein: 18.5g

Steak and Mushroom Noodles

Preparation time: 10 minutes
Cooking time: 20 minutes
Servings: 4

Ingredients:

100g shitake mushrooms, halved, if large

100g chestnut mushrooms, sliced

150g udon noodles

75g kale, finely chopped

75g baby leaf spinach, chopped

2 sirloin steaks

2 teaspoons miso paste

2.5cm piece fresh ginger, finely chopped

2 teaspoons olive oil

1 star anise

1 red chili, finely sliced

1 red onion, finely chopped

1 fresh coriander (cilantro) chopped

1 liter (1½ pints) warm water

Directions:

Pour the water into a saucepan and add in the miso, star anise and ginger. Bring it to the boil, reduce the heat and simmer gently. In the meantime, cook the noodles according to their instructions then drain them.

Heat the oil in a saucepan, add the steak and cook for around 2-3 minutes on each side (or 1-2 minutes, for rare meat).

Remove the meat and set aside.

Place the mushrooms, spinach, coriander (cilantro) and kale into the miso broth and cook for 5 minutes.

In the meantime, heat the remaining oil in a separate pan and fry the chili and onion for 4 minutes, until softened.

Serve the noodles into bowls and pour the soup on top.

Thinly slice the steaks and add them to the top. Serve immediately.

Nutrition:

Calories: 296

Net carbs: 24.6g

Fat: 13.7g

Fiber: 0.7g

Protein: 32.9g

Masala Scallops

Preparation time: 10 minutes
Cooking time: 20 minutes
Servings: 4

Ingredients:

2 tablespoons olive oil

2 jalapenos, chopped

1 pound sea scallops

A pinch of salt and black pepper

¼ teaspoon cinnamon powder

1 teaspoon garam masala

1 teaspoon coriander, ground

1 teaspoon cumin, ground

2 tablespoons cilantro, chopped

Directions:

Heat up a pan with the oil over medium heat, add the jalapenos, cinnamon and the other ingredients except the scallops and cook for 10 minutes.

Add the rest of the ingredients, toss, cook for 10 minutes more, divide into bowls and serve.

Nutrition:

Calories: 251

Fat: 4g

Fiber: 4g

Carbs: 11g

Protein: 17g

Chapter 3 Dinner Recipes

Fresh Fruit Pizza

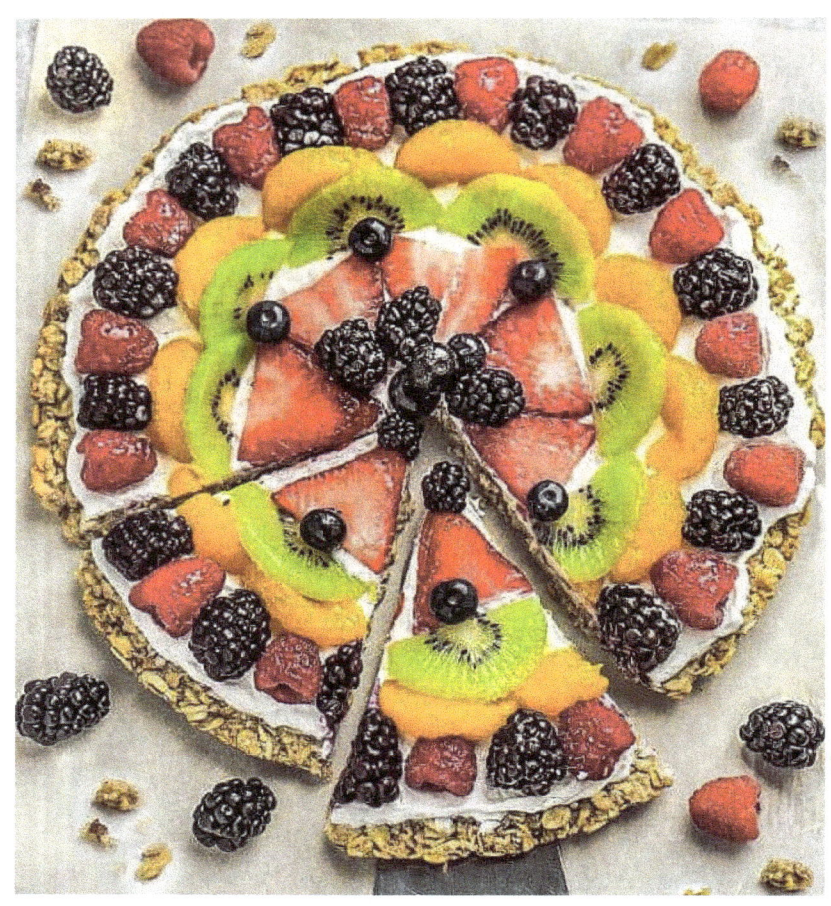

Preparation time: 15 minutes
Cooking time: 14 minutes
Servings: 3

Ingredients:

4 crescent rolls (Rolled-out and poked with a fork)

Two spoonful's of moderate Cream-cheese

Inch teaspoon of sugar

1 teaspoon Vanilla extract

Handful berries - chopped (You Can easily utilize lemon, blueberries or beer)

Sliced almonds

Directions:

Place crescent rolls non-stick pan and then poke a few times with a fork. Cook at 375 for approximately 14 minutes. Let cool.

At a bowl, combine cream, Vanilla infusion & sugar stir with a spoon.

Spread onto crescent rolls, then add almonds and fruit.

I sprinkled a bit more sugar at the top after!

Nutrition:

Calories: 307 Net carbs: 42.8g

Fat: 10.1g Fiber: 2.1g Protein: 10.7g

Apple Blackcurrant Compote Pancakes

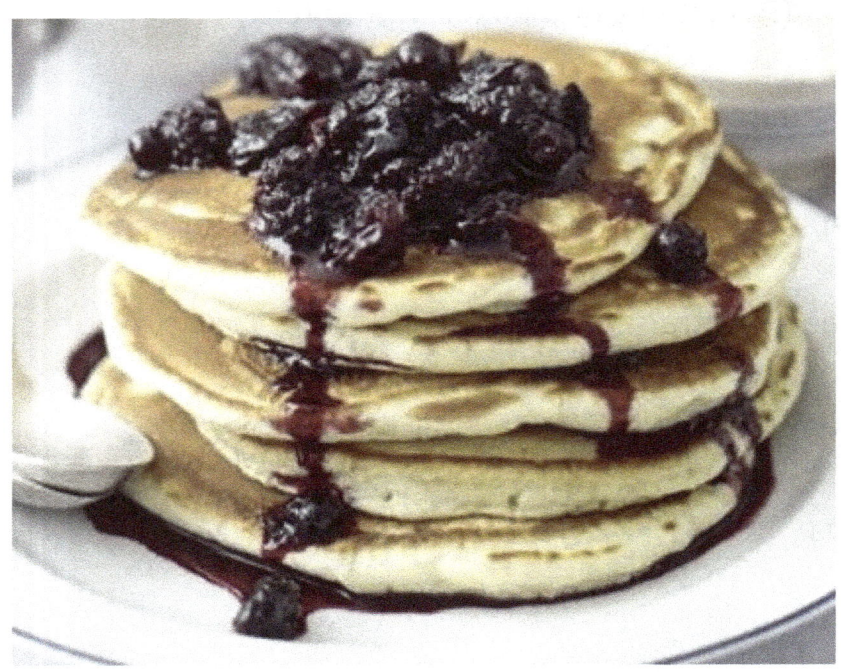

Preparation time: 5 minutes
Cooking time: 15 minutes
Servings: 4

Ingredients:

For the compote:

3s of water 2s caster sugar

120 grams blackcurrants, washed and stalks removed

For The Apple Pancakes:

2 teaspoons light olive oil 2 egg whites 300 ml semi-skimmed milk

2 apples, cut into small pieces

Pinch of salt

2s of caster sugar

1 teaspoon of baking powder

125 grams plain flour

75 grams porridge oats

Directions:

In a small pan, add the blackcurrants, water and sugar. Bring to a gentle boil and let it cook for 10 to 15 minutes.

In a large bowl, place the flour, oats, baking powder, salt and caster sugar, mix well.

Add in the apple, stir and gently fold in semi-skimmed milk until mixture is smooth.

Beat the egg whites until stiff peaks forms then gently whisk into the flour mixture. Pour batter into a jug.

Heat half teaspoon of oil over medium-high heat in a non-stick frying pan. Add about 1/4 of the batter into the pan. Cook pancake until golden brown on both sides. Drizzle the blackcurrant compote.

Nutrition: Calories: 337 Net carbs: 40 g Fat: 9.82g Fiber: 6.2 g Protein: 32g

Blueberry Oats Pancakes

Preparation time: 5 minutes
Cooking time: 5 minutes
Servings: 4

INGREDIENTS:

225 grams blueberries ¼ teaspoon salt 2 teaspoon baking powder

150 grams rolled oats 6 eggs 6 bananas

Directions:

Pulse the rolled oats for 1 minute in a (dry) high-speed blender to form oat flour.

Add in the eggs, bananas, salt and baking powder and process for 2 minutes until it forms a smooth batter.

Pour the batter into a large bowl and gently stir in the blueberries. Let sit for at least 10 minutes to activate the baking powder.

Add a large spoonful of butter to the frying pan over a medium high heat. Scoop the batter and cook until nicely golden underneath. Flip pancake and cook the other side.

Nutrition:

Calories: 494 Net carbs: 68 g Fat: 11.3g Fiber: 6.2 g Protein: 22.23g

Muesli Yoghurt Breakfast

Preparation time: 3 minutes
Cooking time: 0 minutes
Servings: 1

INGREDIENTS:

100g plain Greek, coconut or soya yoghurt

100g hulled and chopped strawberries

10g cocoa nibs

15g chopped walnuts

40g pitted and chopped Medjool dates

15g coconut flakes

10g buckwheat puffs

20g buckwheat flakes

Directions:

Mix together the cocoa nibs, buckwheat flakes, coconut flakes, buckwheat puffs, Medjool dates and walnuts. Add the yoghurt and strawberries.

Nutrition:

Calories: 368 Net carbs: 49g Fat: 11.5g Fiber: 7.4g Protein: 16.54g

Omelette Fold

Preparation time: 3 minutes
Cooking time: 5 minutes
Servings: 1

INGREDIENTS:

1 teaspoon extra virgin olive oil

5 grams thinly sliced parsley 35 grams thinly sliced red chicory

3 medium eggs

50 grams streaky bacon, cut into thin strips

Directions:

Cook the bacon strips in hot non-stick frying pan over high heat until crispy. Remove and drain any excess fat on a kitchen paper.

Beat the eggs in a small bowl and mix with the parsley and chicory. Mix the drained bacon through the egg mixture.

Heat the olive oil in a non-stick pan; add the mixture. Cook until omelette is set. Loose the omelette around the edges with a spatula and fold into half-moon.

Nutrition:

Calories: 471 Net carbs: 3.3g Fat: 38.72g Fiber: 1.5g Protein: 27g

Sticky Chicken Water Melon Noodle Salad

Preparation time: 15 minutes
Cooking time: 25 minutes
Servings: 3

Ingredients:

2 pieces of skinny rice noodles

1/2 tablespoon sesame oil

2 cups Water Melon

Head of bib lettuce

Half of a Lot of scallions

Half of a Lot of fresh cilantro

2 skinless, boneless chicken breasts

1/2 Tablespoon Chinese five-spice

1 tablespoon extra-virgin olive oil

Two tablespoon sweet skillet

1 tablespoon sesame seeds

A couple of cashews - smashed

Dressing - could be made daily or 2 until

1 tablespoon low-salt soy sauce

1 teaspoon sesame oil

1 tablespoon peanut butter

Half of a refreshing red chili

Half of a couple of chives

Half of a couple of cilantro

Inch limes - juiced

1 small spoonful of garlic

Directions:

At a bowl, then completely substituting the noodles in boiling drinking water. They are going to be soon carried out in 2 minutes.

On a big sheet of parchment paper, then throw the chicken with pepper, salt, and also the five-spice.

Twist over the newspaper, subsequently celebration and put the chicken using a rolling pin.

Place into the large skillet with 1 tablespoon of olive oil, turning 3 or 4 minutes, until well charred and cooked through.

Drain the noodles and toss with 1 Tablespoon of sesame oil onto a sizable serving dish.

Place 50% the noodles into the moderate skillet, stirring frequently until crispy and nice.

Eliminate the Watermelon skin, then slice the flesh to inconsistent balls and then increase the platter.

Reduce the lettuces and cut into small wedges and also half of a whole lot of leafy greens and scatter the dish.

Place another 1 / 2 the cilantro pack, the soy sauce, coriander, chives, peanut butter, and a dab of water, 1 teaspoon of sesame oil, and the lime juice then mix till smooth.

Set the chicken back to heat, garnish with all the sweet skillet (or my walnut syrup mixture), and toss with the sesame seeds.

Pour the dressing on the salad toss gently with fresh fingers until well coated, then add crispy noodles and then smashed cashews.

Blend chicken pieces and add them to the salad.

Nutrition:

Calories: 318

Net carbs: 17.5g

Fat: 11.8g

Fiber: 3g

Protein: 34.8g

Asian Shrimp Stir-Fry with Buckwheat Noodles

Preparation time: 15 minutes
Cooking time: 15 minutes
Servings: 1

Ingredients:

150g shelled raw jumbo shrimp, deveined

2 teaspoons tamari

2 teaspoons extra virgin olive oil

75g soba (buckwheat noodles)

2 garlic cloves, chopped

1 Thai chili, chopped

1 teaspoon chopped fresh ginger

20g red onions, sliced

45g celery including leaves, trimmed and cut, with leaves mounted.

Directions:

Load the shrimp onto a tray. Wipe the pan out with a towel of ink, because you will be using it again. Cook the noodles for 5 to 8 minutes in boiling water, or as indicated on the box. Drain and put away. Meanwhile, in the remaining tamari and oil over medium-high heat, fry the garlic, chili, ginger, red onion, celery (but not the leaves), green beans, and kale for 2 to 3 min. Add the stock and allow to a boil, then cook for a minute or two until cooked but crunchy. Add the shrimp, noodles, and leaves of celery to the pan, bring back to a boil, then remove and serve from heat.

Nutrition: Calories: 288 Fat: 21.5g Protein: 22.9g

Miso and Sesame Glazed Tofu with Ginger and Chili Stir-Fried Greens

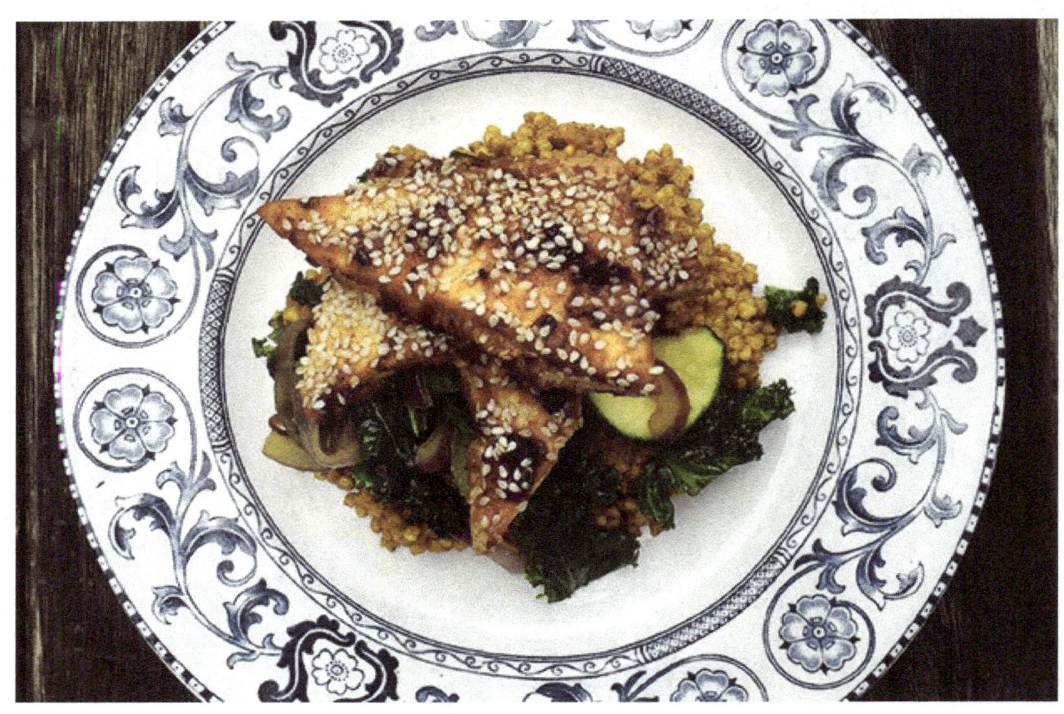

Preparation time: 20 minutes
Cooking time: 45 minutes
Servings: 4

Ingredients:

1 mirin

20gmiso paste

150g block of ram tofu

40g celery

40g red onion, sliced

120g

1 Thai chili

2 garlic cloves

1 teaspoon of nicely chopped fresh ginger

50g kale, chopped

2 teaspoon sesame seeds

35g buckwheat

1 teaspoon ground turmeric

1 teaspoon extra virgin olive oil

1 teaspoon tamari

Directions:

Heat the oven to 400 F. Line a thin, parchment-paper roasting pan.

Mix in the mirin and the miso. Lengthwise cut the tofu, then diagonally cut each piece into triangles in half. Fill the tofu with the miso mix and leave to marinate while the other ingredients are prepared.

Slice the angle into the celery, red onion, and zucchini. Chop the chili, garlic, and ginger thinly, then set aside.

Let the Kale for 5 minutes in a steamer. Discard and set aside.

Place the tofu in the roasting pan, sprinkle the tofu with the sesame seeds, and roast in the oven for 15 to 20 minutes until it has been beautifully caramelized.

Wash the buckwheat in a sieve, then place it along with the turmeric in a saucepan of boiling water. Cook as indicated by a box, then drain.

Heat the oil in a frying pan; add the celery, onion, zucchini, chili, garlic, and ginger and fry over high heat for 1 to 2 minutes, then reduce to medium heat for 3 to 4 minutes until the vegetables are cooked through, but are still crunchy. If the vegetables begin to stick to the pan, you can need to add a cup of water. Add the tamari and kale, and cook for another minute.

Serve with the greens and buckwheat, when the tofu is finished.

Nutrition:

Calories: 547

Net carbs: 72.7g

Fat: 16.5g

Fiber: 14.8g

Protein: 32.1g

Kale and Red Onion Dal with Buckwheat

Preparation time: 10 minutes
Cooking time: 15 minutes
Servings: 1

Ingredients:

1 teaspoon of extra virgin olive oil

1 teaspoon of mustard seeds

40g of red onion, nicely chopped

2 garlic cloves, nicely chopped

1 teaspoon of nicely chopped fresh ginger

1 Thai chili, nicely chopped

1 teaspoon of mild curry powder (medium or soft, if you prefer)

2 teaspoons of ground turmeric

300ml vegetable stock or water

40 g) red lentils, rinsed

50g kale, chopped

Directions:

By the time the mustard seeds start popping, add the onion, garlic, ginger, and chili. Cook until tender, for about 10 minutes.

Add the turmeric curry powder and 1 teaspoon, and cook the spices for a few minutes. Stir in the stock and bring to a boil. Add the lentils to the saucepan and simmer for another 25 to 30 minutes until the lentils are cooked through, and a smooth dal is present.

Add milk to the kale and coconut and cook for another 5 minutes.

In the meantime, cook the buckwheat with the remaining turmeric teaspoon, as per the package instructions. Drain alongside the dal and serve.

Nutrition:

Calories: 72 Net carbs: 6.8g

Fat: 4.3g Fiber: 2.6g Protein: 3.6g

Lamb, Butternut Squash and Date Tagine

Preparation time: 5 minutes
Cooking time: 1 Hour 15 minutes
Servings: 4

Ingredients: 2 tablespoons coconut oil

1 Red onion, chopped

2cm ginger, grated

3 Garlic cloves, crushed or grated

1 teaspoon chili flakes (or to taste)

2 tablespoon cumin seeds

2 teaspoons ground turmeric

1 cinnamon stick

800g lamb neck fillet, cut into 2cm chunks

1/2 tablespoon salt

100g Medjool dates, pitted and sliced

400g Tin chopped berries, and half of a can of plain water

500g Butternut squash, chopped into 1cm cubes

400g Tin chickpeas, drained

2 tablespoons fresh coriander (and extra for garnish)

Buckwheat, Couscous, flatbread or rice to function

Directions:

Pre Heat Your oven to 140C.

Drizzle Roughly 2 tablespoons of coconut oil into a large ovenproof saucepan or cast-iron casserole dish. Add the chopped onion and cook on a gentle heat, with the lid for around five minutes, until the onions are softened but not too brown.

Insert The grated ginger and garlic, chili, cumin, cinnamon, and garlic. Stir well and cook 1 minute with off the lid. Add a dash of water when it becomes too humid.

Next, A DD from the lamb balls. Stir to coat the beef from the spices and onions, then add the salt chopped meats and berries and roughly half of a can of plain water (100-200ml).

Bring the tagine into the boil and put the lid and put on your skillet for about 1 hour and fifteen minutes.

Ten Moments prior to the conclusion of this cooking period, add the chopped butternut squash and drained chickpeas. Stir everything together, place the lid back and go back to the oven to the last half an hour of cooking.

When that is done, the tagine is able to remove from the oven and then stir fry throughout the chopped coriander. Drink buckwheat, couscous, flatbread, or basmati rice.

Nutrition: Calories: 82 Net carbs: 21.5g

Fat: 0.1g Protein: 1.8g

Turmeric Baked Salmon

Preparation time: 10 -- 1-5 moments
Cooking time: 10 Moments
Servings: 1

Ingredients:

150g skinned Salmon

1 teaspoon extra virgin coconut oil

1 teaspoon Ground turmeric

1/4 Juice of a lemon

To get the hot celery

1 teaspoon extra virgin coconut oil

40g Red onion, finely chopped

60g Tinned green peas

1 garlic clove, finely chopped

1cm fresh ginger, finely chopped

1 Bird's eye chili, finely chopped

150g Celery, cut into 2cm lengths

1 teaspoon darkened curry powder

130g Tomato, cut into 8 wedges

100mk vegetable or pasta stock

1 tablespoon parsley, chopped

Directions:

Heat the oven to 200C / gas mark 6.

Start using the hot celery. Heat a skillet over a moderate --low heat, then add the olive oil then the garlic, onion, ginger, celery, and peppermint. Fry lightly for two-three minutes until softened but not colored, you can add the curry powder and cook for a further minute.

Insert the berries afterward, your lentils and stock, and simmer for 10 seconds. You might choose to increase or reduce the cooking time according to how crunchy you'd like your own sausage.

Meanwhile, mix the garlic olive oil and lemon juice and then rub the salmon.

Set on the baking dish and cook 8--10 seconds.

In order to complete, stir the skillet throughout the celery and function with the salmon.

Nutrition:

Calories: 39

Net carbs: 0.1g

Fat: 1.7g

Protein: 5.5g

Coconut and Quinoa Banana Pudding

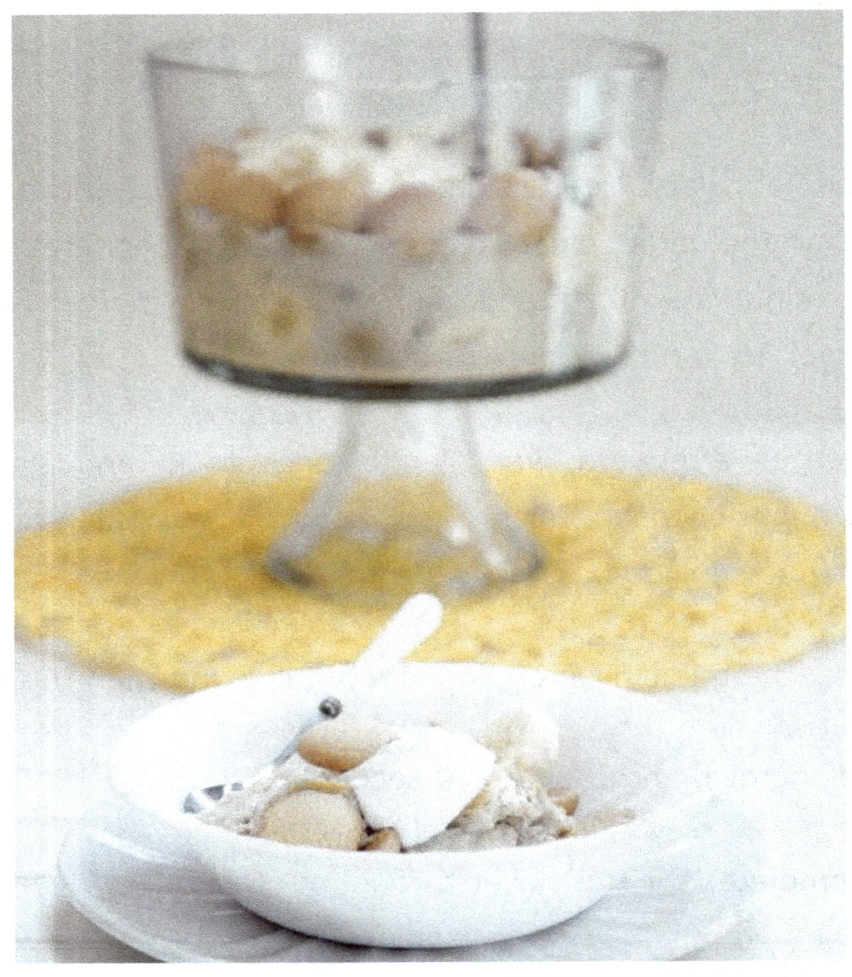

Preparation time: 5 minutes
Cooking time: 30 minutes
Servings: 3

Ingredients:

1 cup quinoa

3 cups coconut milk

3 ripe bananas

¼ cup flaked unsweetened coconut

4 teaspoons sugar

1 teaspoon vanilla extract

Directions:

Wash and cook quinoa according to package directions.

When ready remove from heat and set aside.

In a separate bowl blend sugar, milk and bananas until smooth.

Add to the quinoa.

Heat over medium heat, string, until creamy.

Stir in vanilla and coconut flakes and serve warm.

Nutrition:

Calories: 29

Net carbs: 5.2g

Fat: 0.4g Protein: 0.8g

Crunchy Chocolate Chip Coconut Macadamia Nut Cookies

Preparation time: 15 minutes
Cooking time: 5 minutes
Servings: 5

Ingredients:

1 cup yogurt 1 cup yogurt

1/2 teaspoon baking soda

1/2 teaspoon salt

1 of butter, softened

1 cup firmly packed brown sugar

1/2 cup sugar

1 large egg

1/2 cup semi-sweet chocolate chips

1/2 cup sweetened flaked coconut

1/2 cup coarsely chopped dry-roasted macadamia nuts

1/2 cup raisins

Directions:

Preheat the oven to 325ºf.

In a little bowl, whisk together the flour, oats and baking soda and salt; then place aside.

In your mixer bowl, mix together the butter/sugar/egg mix.

Mix in the flour/oats mix until just combined and stir into the chocolate chips, raisins, nuts, and coconut.

Place outsized bits on a parchment-lined cookie sheet.

Bake for 1-3 minutes, before biscuits are only barely golden brown.

Remove from the oven and then leave the cookie sheets to cool at least 10 minutes.

Nutrition:

Calories: 317 Net carbs: 20.5g

Fat: 9.9g Fiber: 2.3g Protein: 35.2g

Peach and Blueberry Pie

Preparation time: 20 minutes
Cooking time: 60 minutes
Servings: 4

Ingredients:

1 box of noodle dough

Filling:

5 peaches, peeled and chopped (I used roasted peaches)

3 cups strawberries

3/4 cup sugar

1/4 cup bread

Juice of 1/2 lemon

1 egg yolk, beaten

Directions:

Preheat oven to 400 degrees.

Place dough to a 9-inch pie plate

In a big bowl, combine tomatoes, sugar, bread, and lemon juice, then toss to combine. Pour into the pie plate, mounding at the center.

Simply take some of bread and then cut into bits, then put a pie shirt and put the dough in addition to pressing on edges.

Brush crust with egg wash then sprinkles with sugar. Set onto a parchment paper-lined baking sheet. Bake at 400 for about 20 minutes, until crust is browned at borders.

Turn oven down to 350, bake for another 40 minutes. Remove and let sit at least 30minutes.

Have with vanilla ice-cream.

Nutrition:

Calories: 360 Net carbs: 49.2g

Fat: 17.4g Protein: 3.9g

Chicken with Kale and Chili Salsa

Preparation time: 5 minutes
Cooking time: 40 minutes
Servings: 3

Ingredients:

50g of buckwheat

1 teaspoon of chopped fresh ginger

Juice of ½ lemon, divided

2 teaspoon ground turmeric

50g kale, chopped

20g red onion, sliced

120g skinless, boneless chicken breast

1teaspoon extra virgin olive oil

1 tomato

1 handful parsley

1 bird's eye chili, chopped

Directions:

Start with the salsa: remove the eye out of the tomato and finely chop it, making sure to keep as much of the liquid as you can.

Mix it with the chili, parsley, and lemon juice.

You could add everything to a blender for different results.

Heat your oven to 220F.

Marinate the chicken with a little oil, 1 teaspoon of turmeric, and the lemon juice.

Let it rest for 5-10 minutes.

Heat a pan over medium heat until it is hot then add marinated chicken and allow it to cook for a minute on both sides until it is pale gold).

Transfer the chicken to the oven (if pan is not ovenproof place it in a baking tray) and bake for 8 to 10 minutes or until it is cooked through.

Take the chicken out of the oven, cover with foil, and let it rest for five minutes before you serve.

Meanwhile, in a steamer, steam the kale for about 5 minutes.

In a little oil, fry the ginger and red onions until they are soft but not colored, and then add in the cooked kale and fry it for a minute.

Cook the buckwheat in accordance to the packet directions with the remaining turmeric.

Serve alongside the vegetables, salsa and chicken.

Nutrition:

Calories: 130

Net carbs: 4.6g

Fat: 3.8g

Fiber: 2.6g

Protein: 82g

Sirt Salmon Salad

Preparation time: 5 minutes
Cooking time: 30 minutes
Servings: 3

Ingredients:

1 large Medjool date, pitted then chopped

50g of chicory leaves 50g of rocket

1 teaspoon of extra virgin olive oil

10g of parsley, chopped

10g of celery leaves, chopped

40g of celery, sliced

15g of walnuts, chopped 1g of capers

20g of red onions-sliced

80g of avocado-peeled, stoned, and sliced

Juice of ¼ lemon

100g of smoked salmon slices (alternatives: lentils, tinned tuna, or cooked chicken breast)

Directions:

Arrange all the salad leaves on a large plate then mix the rest of the ingredients and distribute evenly on top the leaves.

Nutrition: Calories: 353 Net carbs: 28.1g

Fat: 9.8g Fiber: 4.9g Protein: 40.3g

Greek Salad Skewers

Preparation time: 5 minutes
Cooking time: 30 minutes
Servings: 3

Ingredients:

100g of cucumber, cut into 4 slices and halved (about 10cm)

8 cherry tomatoes

100g feta, cut into 8 cubes

8 large black olives

1 yellow pepper, cut into 8 squares

½ red onion, cut in half and separated into 8 pieces

2 wooden skewers, soaked in water for 30 minutes before use

For the dressing:

Juice of ½ lemon

½ garlic clove, peeled and crushed

1 teaspoon of extra virgin olive oil

A few leaves of finely chopped basil

Generous seasoning of salt and freshly ground black pepper a few finely chopped oregano leaves

1 teaspoon of balsamic vinegar

Directions:

Thread every skewer with salad ingredients in this order; olive, followed by tomato, then yellow pepper, red onion, followed by cucumber then feta, tomato, olive, then yellow pepper, red onion and finally cucumber.

Place the dressing ingredients in a small bowl, mix them thoroughly, and then pour over the skewers.

Nutrition:

Calories: 220

Net carbs: 4.4g

Fat: 19.6g

Fiber: 3g

Protein: 7.2g

Alkalizing Green Soup

Preparation time: 5 minutes
Cooking time: 40 minutes
Servings: 3

Ingredients:

2 cups broccoli, cut into florets and chopped

2 zucchinis, peeled and chopped

2 cups chopped kale

1 small onion, chopped

2-3 garlic cloves, chopped

4 cups vegetable broth

2 extra virgin olive oil

½ teaspoon ground ginger

½ teaspoon ground coriander

1 lime, juiced, to serve

Directions:

Gently heat olive oil in a large saucepan over medium-high heat.

Cook onion and garlic for 3-4 minutes until tender.

Add ginger and coriander and stir to coat well.

Add in broccoli, zucchinis, kale and vegetable broth.

Bring to the boil, then reduce heat and simmer for 15 minutes, stirring from time to time.

Set aside to cool and blend until smooth.

Return to pan and cook until heated through. Serve with lime juice.

Nutrition:

Calories: 77

Net carbs: 11.2g

Fat: 2.1g

Fiber: 0.5g

Protein: 3.5g

Creamy Broccoli and Potato Soup

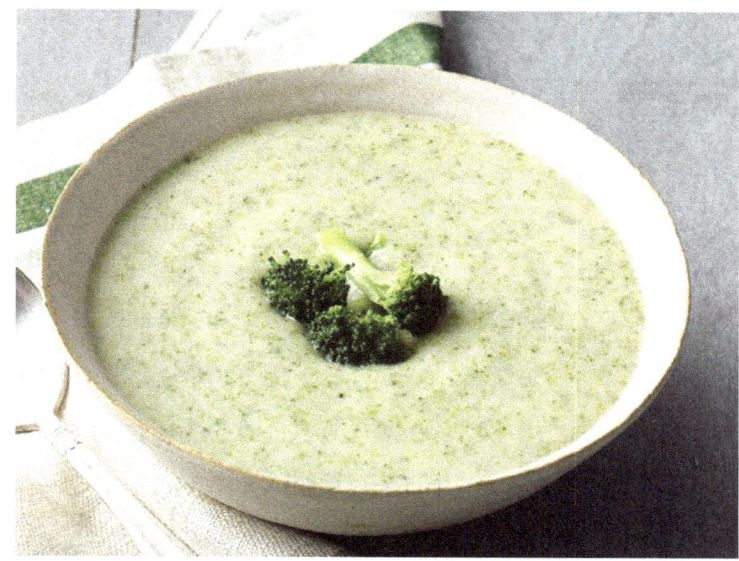

Preparation time: 5 minutes
Cooking time: 30 minutes
Servings: 3

Ingredients:

3 cups broccoli, cut into florets and chopped

2 potatoes, peeled and chopped

1 large onion, chopped

3 garlic cloves, minced

1 cup raw cashews 1 cup vegetable broth

4 cups water

3 teaspoons extra virgin olive oil

½ teaspoon ground nutmeg

Directions:

Soak cashews in a bowl covered with water for at least 4 hours. Drain water and blend cashews with 1 cup of vegetable broth until smooth. Set aside. Gently heat olive oil in a large saucepan over medium-high heat. Cook onion and garlic for 3-4 minutes until tender. Add in broccoli, potato, nutmeg and water.

Cover and bring to the boil, then reduce heat and simmer for 20 minutes, stirring from time to time. Remove from heat and stir in cashew mixture.

Blend until smooth, return to pan and cook until heated through.

Nutrition:

Calories: 105 Net carbs: 14.2g Fat: 3.5g

Fiber: 0.5g Protein: 3.7g

Creamy Brussels Sprout Soup

Preparation time: 5 minutes
Cooking time: 35 minutes
Servings: 3

Ingredients: 1 large onion, chopped

1lb frozen Brussels sprouts, thawed

2 potatoes, peeled and chopped

3 garlic cloves, minced

1 cup raw cashews

4 cups vegetable broth

3 teaspoons extra virgin olive oil

½ teaspoon curry powder

Salt and black pepper, to taste

Directions:

Soak cashews in a bowl covered with water for at least 4 hours. rain water and blend cashews with 1 cup of vegetable broth until smooth. Set aside. Gently heat olive oil in a large saucepan over medium-high heat.

Cook onion and garlic and for 3-4 minutes until tender.

Add in Brussels sprouts, potato, curry and vegetable broth.

Cover and bring to a boil, then reduce heat and simmer for 20 minutes, stirring from time to time.

Remove from heat and stir in cashew mixture. Blend until smooth, return to pan and cook until heated through.

Nutrition: Calories: 38 Net carbs: 7.8g

Fat: 0.2g Protein: 2.9g

Chapter 4 Snacks

Lemongrass Green Tea

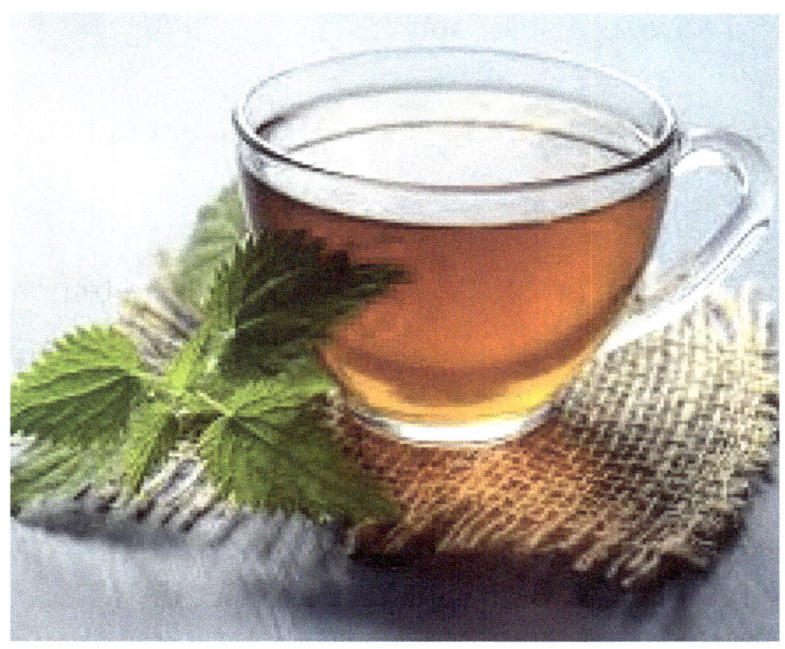

Preparation time: 3 minutes
Cooking time: 12 min
Servings: 1

Ingredients:

Two teaspoons cleaved lemongrass

One teaspoon green tea leaves

1 cup of water

One teaspoon nectar

Directions:

Move the water to a treated steel pot.

Hurl in the lemongrass and heat the water to the point of boiling. Let it bubble for 5 minutes.

Expel the pot from the fire and let the water cool till the temperature is 80-85 degrees C.

Presently, include the green tea and let it soak for 3 minutes.

Strain the tea into your cup.

Include nectar and mix a long time before drinking.

Nutrition:

Calories: 2.5 Calcium: 3mg

Potassium: 34mg Magnesium: 2.9g

Grape and Melon Juice

Preparation time: 10 minutes
Cooking time: 0 minutes
Servings: 1

Ingredients:

½ cucumber, stripped whenever liked, split, seeds evacuated and generally slashed

30g youthful spinach leaves stalks expelled

100g red seedless grapes

100g melon, stripped, deseeded

Directions:

Cut into pieces. Blend in a juicer or blender until smooth.

Nutrition:

Calories: 125

Net carbs: 31.7g

Fat: 0.24g

Protein: 0.63g

Kale and Blackcurrant Smoothie

Preparation time: 10 minutes
Cooking time: 0 minutes
Servings: 2

Ingredients:

2 teaspoon nectar

1 cup crisply made green tea

Ten infant kale leaves stalk expelled

One ready banana

40 g blackcurrants, washed and stalks evacuated

Six ice blocks

Directions:

Mix the nectar into the warm green tea until disintegrated. Master all the fixings together in a blender until smooth. Serve right away.

Nutrition:

Calories: 86

Net carbs: 32.9g

Protein: 4.5g

Kale, Edamame and Tofu Curry

Preparation time: 5 minutes
Cooking time: 8 minutes
Servings: 4

Ingredients:

1 teaspoon rapeseed oil

One huge onion, cleaved

Four cloves garlic stripped and ground

One massive thumb (7cm) crisp ginger, stripped and ground

One red bean stew, deseeded and meagerly cut

1/2 teaspoon ground turmeric

1/4 teaspoon cayenne pepper

1 teaspoon paprika 1 teaspoon salt

1/2 teaspoon ground cumin

250g dried red lentils 1-litre bubbling water

50g solidified soy edamame beans

200g firm tofu, cleaved into solid shapes

Two tomatoes, generally cleaved

Juice of 1 lime

200g kale leaves stalks expelled and torn

Directions:

Put the oil in an overwhelming bottomed container over a low-medium warmth. Include the onion and cook for 5 minutes before including the garlic, ginger and stew and preparing for a further 2 minutes. Include the turmeric, cayenne, paprika, cumin and salt. Mix through before including the red lentils and blending once more.

pour in the bubbling water and bring to a generous stew for 10 minutes, at that point decrease the warmth and cook for a further 20-30 minutes until the curry has a thick '•porridge' consistency.

Add the soya beans, tofu and tomatoes and cook for a further 5 minutes. Include the lime juice and kale leaves and cook until the kale merely is delicate.

Nutrition: Protein: 12.6g

Calories: 342 Net carbs: 8.4g Fat: 17g

Lemongrass Green Tea

Preparation time: 10 minutes
Cooking time: 0 minutes
Servings: 2

Ingredients:

Two ready bananas 250 ml of milk

2 teaspoon matcha green tea powder

1/2 teaspoon vanilla bean glue (not separate) or a little scratch of the seeds from a vanilla unit

Six ice blocks 2 teaspoon nectar

Directions:

Just mix all the fixings in a blender and serve in two glasses.

Nutrition:

Calories: 183 Net carbs: 33g Fat: 0.6g

Fiber: 3.8g Protein: 2.1g

Sirt Muesli

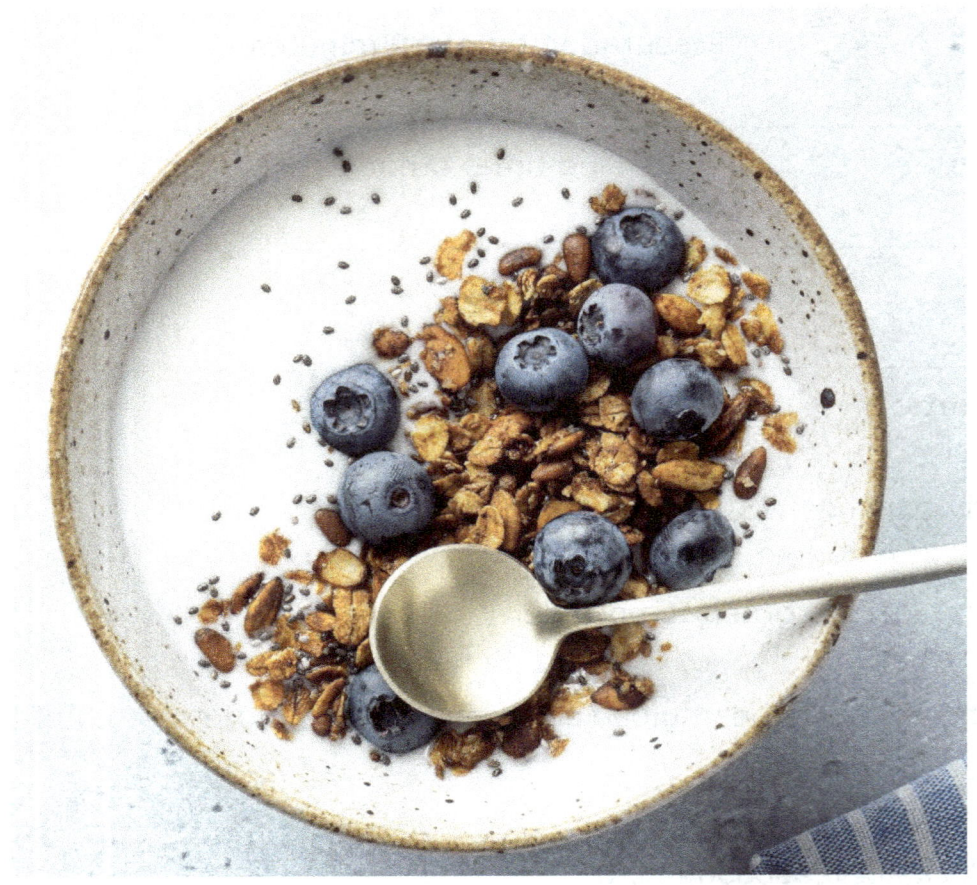

Preparation time: 10 minutes
Cooking time: 0 minutes
Servings: 2

Ingredients:

20g buckwheat flakes sirtfood plans

10g buckwheat puffs

15g parched coconut

40g Medjool dates, hollowed and cleaved

15g pecans, cleaved

10g cocoa nibs

100g strawberries, hulled and cleaved

100g plain Greek yoghurt (or veggie lover elective, for example, soya or coconut yoghurt)

Directions:

Blend the entirety of the above fixings, possibly including the yoghurt and strawberries before serving on the off chance that you are making it in mass.

Nutrition:

Calories: 25

Net carbs: 43.3g

Fat: 7.2g

Fiber: 6.5g

Protein: 9.0g

Fruit Salad

Preparation time: 10 min
Cooking time: 0 minutes
Servings: 1

Ingredients:

½ cup crisply made green tea

1 teaspoon nectar One orange, split

One apple, cored and generally cleaved

Ten red seedless grapes

Ten blueberries

Directions:

Stir the nectar into a large portion of some green tea. At the point when broken up, include the juice of a large part of the orange. Leave to cool.

Chop the other portion of the orange and spot in a bowl together with the hacked apple, grapes and blueberries. Pour over the cooled tea and leave to soak for a couple of moments before serving.

Nutrition: Calories: 157 Net carbs: 13g

Fiber: 1g Protein: 0.5g

Golden Turmeric Latte

Preparation time: 3 minutes
Cooking time: 7 minutes
Servings: 3

Ingredients:

3 cups of coconut milk

One teaspoon turmeric powder

One teaspoon cinnamon powder

One teaspoon crude nectar

Directions:

Spot of dark pepper (expands retention)

Modest bit of new stripped ginger root

Place of cayenne pepper (discretionary)

Mix all fixings in a fast blender until smooth.

Fill a little container and warmth for 4 minutes over medium heat until hot however not bubbling.

Nutrition:

Calories: 50

Net carbs: 98g

Fat: 2.7g

The Sirt Juice

Preparation time: 7-8 min
Cooking time: 0 minutes
Servings: 2

Ingredients:

Two huge bunches (75g) kale

A huge bunch (30g) rocket

A tiny bunch (5g) level leaf parsley

A small bunch (5g) lovage leaves (discretionary)

2–3 huge stalks (150g) green celery, including its leaves

½ medium green apple

Juice of ½ lemon

½ level teaspoon matcha green tea

Directions:

Blend the greens (kale, rocket, parsley and lovage, on the off chance that was utilizing), at that point juice them. We discover juicers can indeed vary in their effectiveness at squeezing verdant vegetables, and you may need to re-squeeze the leftovers before proceeding onward to different fixings. The objective is to wind up with about 50ml of juice from the greens.

Presently squeeze the celery and apple. You can strip the lemon and put it through the juicer also, however, we think that it's a lot simpler just to crush the lemon by hand into the juice. By this stage, you ought to have around 250ml of milk altogether, maybe marginally more. It is just when the sauce is made and prepared to serve that you include the matcha green tea.

Pour a limited quantity of the juice into a glass, at that point include the matcha and mix enthusiastically with a fork or teaspoon. We just use matcha in the first two beverages of the day as it contains reasonable measures of caffeine (a similar substance as a typical cup of tea). For individuals not accustomed to it, it might keep them wakeful whenever alcoholic late once the match is broken up, including the rest of the juice.

Give it a last mix; at that point, your juice is prepared to drink. Don't hesitate to top up with plain water, as indicated by taste.

Nutrition:

Calories: 75

Net carbs: 3.8g

Fat: 0.6g

Fiber: 2.9g

Protein: 0.4g

Kale Pesto Hummus

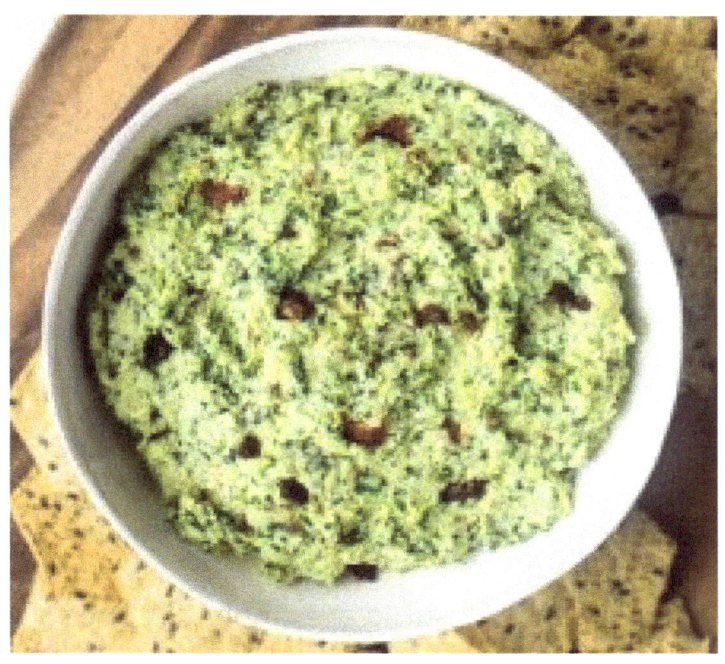

Preparation time: 10 minutes
Cooking time: 7 minutes
Servings: 12

Ingredients:

Chickpeas, drained and liquid reserved – 15 ounces

Reserved chickpea liquid - .25 cup

Sea salt - .5 teaspoon

Tahini paste - .5 cup

Garlic, minced – 2 cloves

Lemon juice – 2.5 s

Extra virgin olive oil - .33 cup

Black pepper, ground - .5 teaspoon

Kale, chopped and leaves packed – 2 cups

Pine nuts – 2 s

Basil leaves, packed – 1.25 cups

Garlic, minced – 4 cloves

Extra virgin olive oil - .25 cup

Directions:

Into a food processor add the basil, kale, pine nuts, and four cloves of minced garlic. Pulse until the leaves and garlic are finely chopped.

Pour in the olive oil, and once again pulse until smooth. Remove the pesto from the bowl of the food processor and set aside.

Into the empty food processor add the remaining ingredients to assemble the hummus, pulsing until creamy. Add in the prepared pesto, and pulse just until the two are combined.

Transfer the pesto hummus to a serving bowl or store in the fridge.

Nutrition:

Calories: 194 Net carbs: 3.8g

Fat: 2.2g Fiber: 1.8g Protein: 5.6g

Parsley Hummus

Preparation time: 5 minutes
Cooking time: 7 minutes
Servings: 6

Ingredients:

Chickpeas, drained and rinsed – 15 ounces

Curly parsley, stems removed – 1 cup

Sea salt – .5 teaspoon

Soy milk, unsweetened - .5 cup

Extra virgin olive oil – 3 teaspoons

Lime juice – 1 s

Red pepper flakes -.5 teaspoons

Black pepper, ground - .25 teaspoon

Pine nuts – 2 s

Sesame seeds, toasted – 2 s

Directions:

In the food processor pulse the parsley and toasted sesame seeds until it forms a fine powdery texture. Drizzle in the extra virgin olive oil in while you continue to pulse, until it is smooth.

Add the chickpeas, lime juice, and seasonings to the food processor and pulse while slowly adding in the soy milk. Continue to pulse the parsley hummus until it is smooth and creamy.

Adjust the seasonings to your preference and then serve or refrigerate the hummus.

Nutrition: Calories: 107 Net carbs: 7.7g

Fat: 4.5g Fiber: 0.2g Protein: 8.6g

Edamame Hummus

Preparation time: 7 minutes
Cooking time: 0 minutes
Servings: 10

Ingredients:

Edamame, cooked and shelled – 2 cups

Sea salt – 1 teaspoon

Extra virgin olive oil – 1

Tahini paste - .25 cup

Lemon juice - .25 cup

Garlic, minced – 3 cloves

Black pepper, ground - .25 teaspoon

Directions:

Add the cooked edamame and remaining ingredients to a blender or food processor and mix on high until it forms a creamy and completely smooth mixture. Taste it and adjust the seasonings to your preference.

Serve the hummus immediately with your favorite vegetables or store in the fridge.

Nutrition:

Calories: 88

Net carbs: 3.8g

Protein: 2.6g

Edamame Guacamole

Preparation time: 7 minutes
Cooking time: 0 minutes
Servings: 6

Ingredients:

Edamame, cooked and shelled – 1 cup

Avocado, pitted and halved – 1

Red onion, diced - .5 cup

Cilantro, chopped - .25 cup

Jalapeno, minced – 1

Garlic, minced – 2 cloves

Lime juice – 2 s Water – 3 s

Lime zest - .5 teaspoon

Roma tomato, diced – 2

Cumin - .125 teaspoon

Sea salt - .5 teaspoon

Directions:

Into a blender or food processor add all of the ingredients, except for the diced tomato, onion, and jalapeno. Blend the tomato mixture on high speed until it is smooth and creamy, making sure that the edamame has been completely blended.

Adjust the seasoning to your preference and then transfer the guacamole to a serving bowl. Stir in the tomato, onion, and jalapeno. Place the bowl in the fridge, allowing it to chill for at least thirty minutes before serving.

Nutrition: Calories: 100 Net carbs: 13g

Fat: 6.6g Fiber: 6.2g Protein: 45g

Eggplant Fries with Fresh Aioli

Preparation time: 10 minutes
Cooking time: 25 minutes
Servings: 4

Ingredients:

Eggplants – 2

Black pepper, ground - .25 teaspoon

Extra virgin olive oil – 2 s

Cornstarch – 1

Basil, dried – 1 teaspoon

Garlic powder - .25 teaspoon

Sea salt - .5 teaspoon

Mayonnaise, made with olive oil - .5 cup

Garlic, minced – 1 teaspoon

Basil, fresh, chopped – 1

Lemon juice – 1 teaspoon

Chipotle, ground - .5 teaspoon

Sea salt - .25 teaspoon

Directions:

Begin by preheating your oven to Fahrenheit four-hundred and twenty-five degrees. Place a wire cooking/cooling rack on a baking sheet.

Remove the peel from the eggplants and then slice them into rounds, each about three-quarters of an inch thick. Slice the rounds into wedges one inch in width.

Add the eggplant wedges to a large bowl and toss them with the olive oil. Once coated, add the pepper, cornstarch, dried basil, garlic powder, and sea salt, tossing until evenly coated.

Arrange the eggplant wedges on top of the wire rack and set the baking sheet in the oven, allowing the fries to cook for fifteen to twenty minutes.

Meanwhile, prepare the aioli. To do this, add the remaining ingredients into a small bowl and whisk them together to combine. Cover the bowl of aioli and allow it to chill it in the fridge until the fries are ready to be served.

Remove the fries from the oven immediately upon baking, or allow them to cook under the broiler for an additional three to four minutes for extra crispy fries. Serve immediately with the aioli.

Nutrition:

Calories: 243

Net carbs: 12.6g

Fat: 0.5g

Fiber: 13.2g

Protein: 5.3g

Chapter 5 Desserts Recipes

Snowflakes

Preparation time: 15 minutes
Cooking time: 10 minutes
Servings: 1

Ingredients:

Won ton wrappers

Oil to frying

Powdered sugar

Directions:

Cut won ton wrappers just like you'd a snowflake

Heat oil. When hot, add wonton, fry for approximately 30 seconds then flip over.

Drain on a paper towel and dust with powdered sugar.

Nutrition:

Calories: 96

Net carbs: 24.1g

Fat: 0.6g

Fiber: 5.3g

Protein: 2.8

Home-Made Marshmallow Fluff

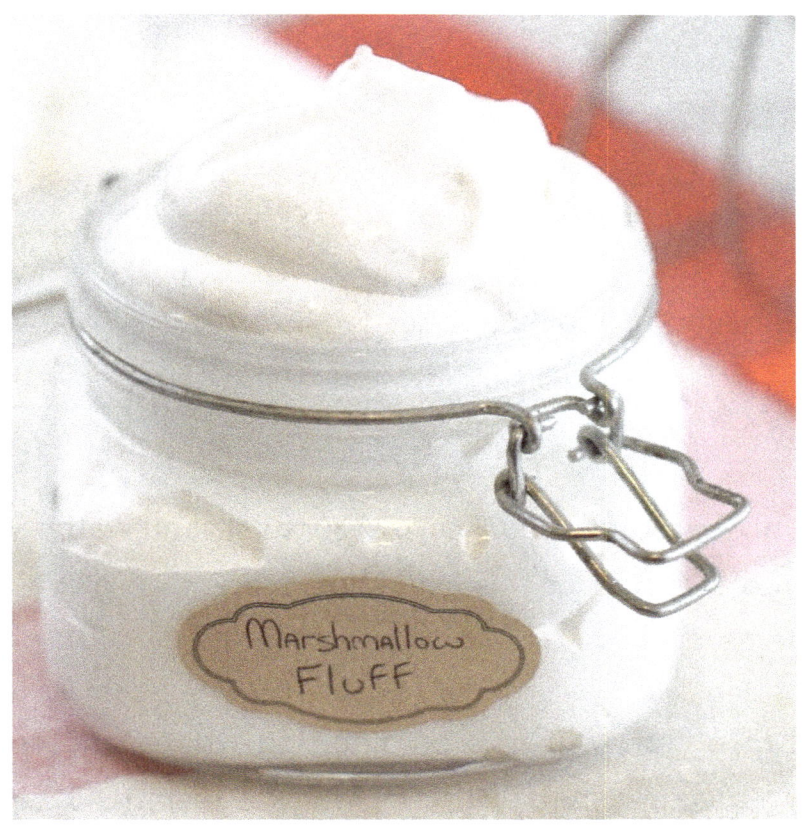

Preparation time: 15 minutes
Cooking time: 20 minutes
Servings: 4

Ingredients:

3/4 cup sugar

1/2 cup light corn syrup

1/4 cup water

⅛ Teaspoon salt

3 little egg whites

1/4 teaspoon cream of tartar

1 teaspoon 1/2 teaspoon vanilla extract

Directions:

In a little pan, mix together sugar, corn syrup, salt and water. Attach a candy thermometer into the side of this pan, but make sure it will not touch the underside of the pan.

From the bowl of a stand mixer, combine egg whites and cream of tartar. Begin to whip on medium speed with the whisk attachment.

Meanwhile, turn a burner on top and place the pan with the sugar mix onto heat. Pout mix into a boil and heat to 240 degrees, stirring periodically.

The aim is to have the egg whites whipped to soft peaks and also the sugar heated to 240 degrees at near the same moment. Simply stop stirring the egg whites once they hit soft peaks.

Once the sugar has already reached 240 amounts, turn heat low allowing it to reduce. Insert a little quantity of the popular sugar mix and let it mix. Insert still another little sum of the sugar mix. Add mix slowly and that means you never scramble the egg whites.

After all of the sugar was added into the egg whites, then decrease the speed of the mixer and also keep mixing concoction for around 7- 9 minutes until the fluff remains glossy and stiff. At roughly the 5-minute mark, then add the vanilla extract.

Use fluff immediately or store in an airtight container in the fridge for around two weeks.

Nutrition:

Calories: 23

Net carbs: 5.8g

Protein: 0.1g

Guilt Totally Free Banana Ice-Cream

Preparation time: 15 minutes
Cooking time: 0 minutes
Servings: 3

Ingredients:

3 quite ripe banana - peeled and chopped

A couple of chocolate chips

Two skim milk

Directions:

Throw all ingredients into a food processor and blend until creamy.

Eat: freeze and appreciate afterward.

Nutrition:

Calories: 387

Net carbs: 47.3g

Fat: 19.5g

Fiber: 1g

Protein: 6.3g

Perfect Little PB Snack Balls

Preparation time: 15 minutes
Cooking time: 0 minutes
Servings: 1

Ingredients:

1/2 cup chunky peanut butter

3 flax seeds

3 wheat germ

1 honey or agave

1/4 cup powdered sugar

Directions:

Blend dry ingredients and adding from the honey and peanut butter.

Mix well and roll into chunks and then conclude by rolling into wheat germ.

Nutrition:

Calories: 95

Net carbs: 6.6g

Fat: 5.6g

Fiber: 1.2g

Protein: 5.7g

Dark Chocolate Pretzel Cookies

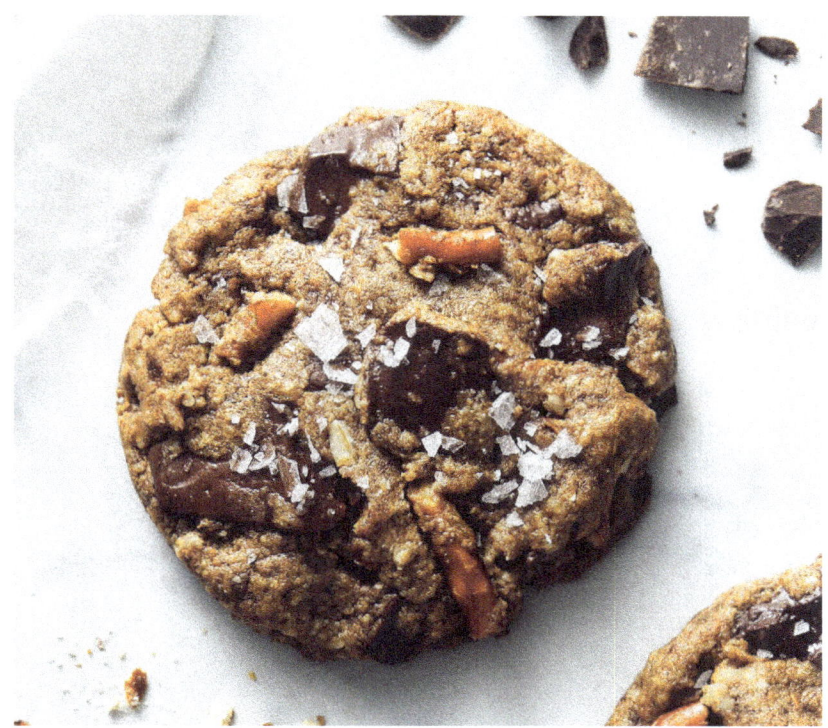

Preparation time: 15 minutes
Cooking time: 20 minutes
Servings: 4

Ingredients:

1 cup yogurt

1/2 teaspoon baking soda

1/4 teaspoon salt

1/4 teaspoon cinnamon

4 butter (softened/0

1/3 cup brown sugar

1 egg

1/2 teaspoon vanilla

1/2 cup dark chocolate chips

1/2 cup pretzels, chopped

Directions:

Preheat oven to 350 degrees.

In a medium bowl whisk together the sugar, butter, vanilla and egg.

In another bowl, stir together the flour, baking soda, and salt.

Stir the bread mixture in, using all the wet components, along with the chocolate chips and pretzels until just blended.

Drop large spoonful of dough on an unlined baking sheet.

Bake for 15-17 minutes, or until the bottoms are somewhat all crispy.

Allow cooling on a wire rack.

Nutrition:

Calories: 300

Net carbs: 44.3g

Fat: 11.2g

Fiber: 1.3g

Protein: 3.8g

Marshmallow Popcorn Balls

Preparation time: 5 minutes
Cooking time: 20 minutes
Servings: 6

Ingredients: 2 bag of microwave popcorn

1 12.6 ounces. Tote M&M's

3 cups honey roasted peanuts

1 pkg. 16 ounce. Massive marshmallows

1 cup butter, cubed

Directions:

In a bowl, blend the popcorn, peanuts and M&M's. In a big pot, combine marshmallows and butter. Cook using medium-low heat. Insert popcorn mix, blend thoroughly Spray muffin tins with non-stick cooking spray.

When cool enough to handle, spray hands together with non-stick cooking spray and then shape into chunks and put into the muffin tin to shape. Add Popsicle stick into each chunk and then let cool.

Wrap each serving in vinyl when chilled.

Nutrition:

Calories: 36 Net carbs: 7.4g Fat: 0.2g

Fiber: 0.3g Protein: 0.9g

Home-Made Ice-Cream Drumsticks

Preparation time: 15 minutes
Cooking time: 0 minutes
Servings: 4

Ingredients:

Vanilla ice cream

Two Lindt hazelnut chunks

Magical shell - out chocolate

Sugar levels

Nuts (I mixed crushed peppers and unsalted peanuts)

Parchment paper

Directions:

Soften ice cream and mixing topping - I had two sliced Lindt hazelnut balls.

Fill underside of Magic shell with sugar and nuts and top with ice-cream.

Wrap parchment paper round cone and then fill cone over about 1.5 inches across the cap of the cone (the paper can help to carry its shape).

Sprinkle with magical nuts and shells.

Freeze for about 20 minutes, before the ice cream is eaten.

Nutrition:

Calories: 267

Net carbs: 32.4g Fat: 14.2g Fiber: 0.9g

Protein: 4.6g

Ultimate Chocolate Chip Cookie N' Oreo Fudge Brownie Bar

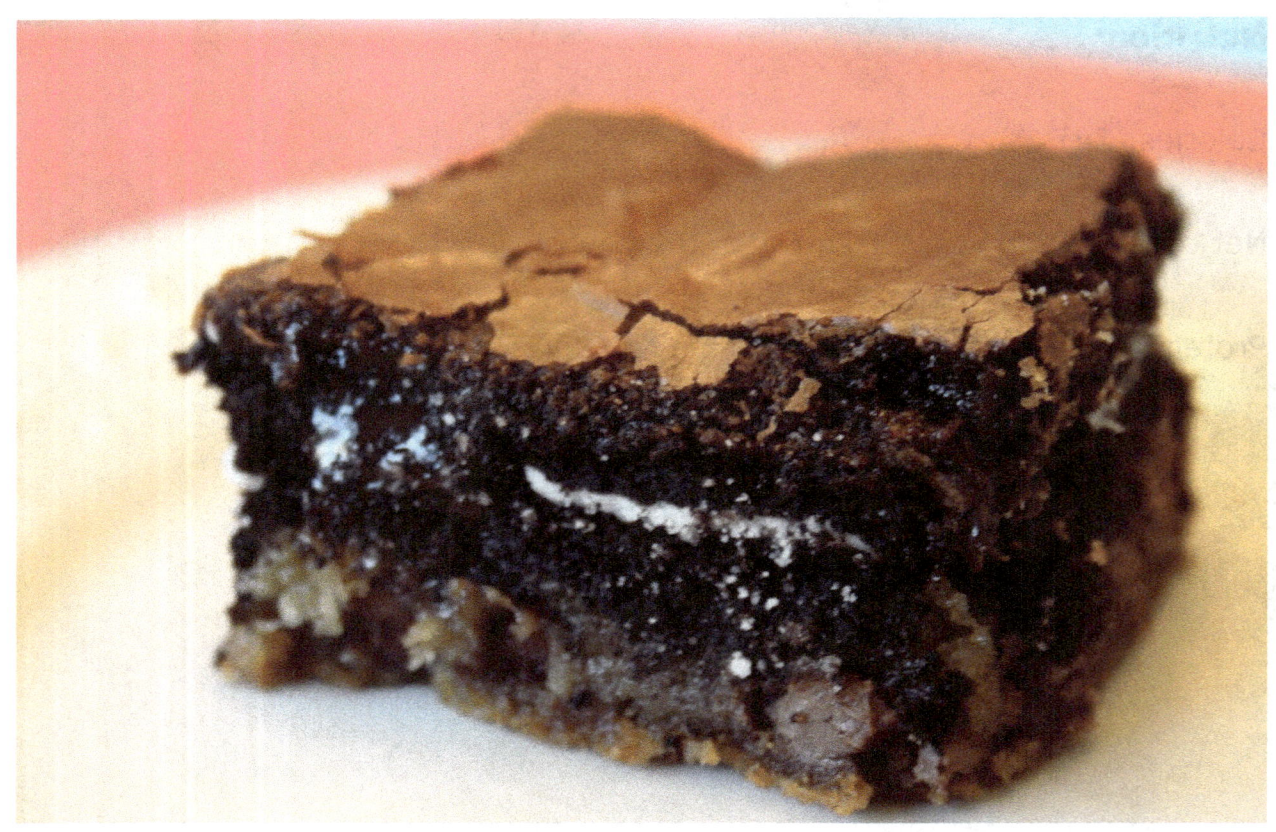

Preparation time: 20 minutes
Cooking time: 70 minutes
Servings: 4

Ingredients:

1 cup (2 sticks) butter, softened

1 cup granulated sugar

3/4 cup light brown sugar

2 large egg

1 pure vanilla extract

2 ½ cups all-purpose flour

1 teaspoon baking soda

1 teaspoon lemon

2 cups (12 Oz) milk chocolate chips

1 package double stuffed Oreo

1 family-size (9×1 3) brownie mixture

1/4 cup hot fudge topping

Directions:

Preheat oven to 350 degrees F.

Cream the butter and sugars in a large bowl using an electric mixer at medium speed for 35 minutes.

Add the vanilla and eggs and mix well to combine thoroughly. In another bowl, whisk together the flour, baking soda and salt, and slowly incorporate in the mixer everything is combined.

Stir in chocolate chips.

Spread the cookie dough at the bottom of a 9×1-3 baking dish that is wrapped with wax paper and then coated with cooking spray.

Shirt with a coating of Oreos. Mix together brownie mix, adding an optional 1/4 cup of hot fudge directly into the mixture.

Stir the brownie batter within the cookie-dough and Oreos.

Cover with foil and bake at 350 degrees F for 30 minutes.

Remove foil and continue baking for another 15 25 minutes.

Let cool before cutting on brownies. They may be gooey at the while warm but will also set up perfectly once chilled.

Nutrition:

Calories: 181

Net carbs: 30g

Fat: 5.4g

Fiber: 1.1g

Protein: 3g

Conclusion

I truly wish you appreciated this experience, thanks for analysis and also attempting these dishes with me.

I advise workout sessions 1 or 2 days a week to shed all the fat well as well as maintain you in leading form.

Make use of these dishes to produce your very own customized consuming strategy to maintain you really feeling excellent.

Hugs and also lengthy real-time sirtfood.

CPSIA information can be obtained
at www.ICGtesting.com
Printed in the USA
LVHW060220240421
685369LV00014B/465

9 781667 160160